UNBREAKABLE

Kyle Zagrodzky, OsteoStrong Founder and CEO

John Jaquish, PhD

Foreword by Tony Robbins

True Wellness, Inc.
8524 Highway 6 North, #310
Houston, Texas 77095

ISBN: 978-1-7352248-1-7

DISCLAIMER

This book is to be used for educational purposes only.

Likewise, any ingredient or health practice, herbal or otherwise, should always be reviewed for safety, as well as contraindications with any current medications with your qualified healthcare provider.

No physical exercise is 100% safe, and neither is OsteoStrong. OsteoStrong provides a unique way to emulate a high impact load of force to achieve osteogenic loading, without the high impact. While not 100% safe, OsteoStrong is significantly safer than attempting high impact force. OsteoStrong members have reported improved bone density, improved balance, improved strength, reduced joint pain, and reduced HbA1c. Results may vary.

It is always advised to consult a medical professional before starting or trying any substance, treatment, exercise, or regimen. Statements in this book have not been evaluated by the FDA and are not intended to diagnose, treat, cure, or prevent any disease or health condition. OsteoStrong centers are independently owned and operated.

John Jaquish received his PhD from Rushmore University, certified/ accredited in accordance with UK National Standards, but whose accreditation is not recognized in some jurisdictions.

Neither the authors nor the publisher accepts any responsibility for the actions of readers of this book.

"Biohack - The philosophical approach of leveraging science and research to develop and apply the most efficient techniques to produce a desired result in physical health."

-Kyle Zagrodzky

FOREWORD

Tony Robbins

For the last four and a half decades, I've been obsessed with finding the things that make a real difference in the quality of peoples' lives. What allows some people to reach new heights of human potential? What are they doing differently?

Whether it's in their relationships, business, emotions, or health, I believe success leaves clues. I've spent a lifetime finding and applying those clues to change my own life, and helping millions of other people do the same.

The term "biohacking" is so overused today that it's almost a cliché. But at the root of it, it's about finding asymmetric risk and reward; the actions you can take that produce the maximum results and benefit, for the smallest amount of time and risk.

If you're here, you're clearly someone that's looking for an edge. You're a forward thinker looking ahead to what hasn't hit the mainstream yet. I deeply admire that drive to go beyond what's known and seek the best technologies available with the power to change the human body and the quality of your life.

The tool you're about to discover is close to my heart because it has not only transformed my life, but also the lives of my wife and my closest family and friends. For me, this tool wasn't just a nice addition to my routine; it was vital.

I have a crazy lifestyle. In a given week I can be in three different countries, visiting different continents, and constantly changing time zones. It's insane! But in every situation, I need to show up and deliver maximum results. To give you an idea, the shortest seminar I normally do is 50 hours, four days and nights.

On a typical event day, I burn approximately 11,300 calories (think of running two marathons) and jump over 1,000 times (the equivalent of two games for an NBA player.) Every jump places four times the normal force of gravity on my body, and on an average day teaching a seminar I was experiencing *a million pounds* of pressure on my body.

A million pounds of pressure! I was shocked to learn this. I'd been doing this for forty years, not knowing what I had been putting my body through.

For me, my bone and structural strength is non-negotiable. If you know anything about me, you know that energy is fundamental to everything I do. You need energy to execute. Energy is where action comes from. Without enormous amounts of energy, power and strength, I wouldn't be able to deliver massive impact.

The good news is, at 60 years old, I'm more active than ever because I have incredible bone strength. And it's not just me; my wife Sage and I both use these technologies.

I'm a fitness and health fanatic, but my wife never used to exercise consistently. Now she's addicted because with the OsteoStrong process you can exercise for a mere ten minutes and produce a maximum amount of increased strength. That's it. Talk about simple to execute! No sweat, no soreness, and each week we get stronger and stronger. I know this sounds impossible, but it's based on proven science.

More importantly, you can test these devices with your own body and see the amazing improvements in strength that happen in just a few weeks. When you're applying precisely the right stimulus to the body, you get an extraordinary result.

We're both hooked. I've dedicated my life to giving people the most value I can possibly generate in the shortest period of time. Why? Because there's something else I've learned that the world's top performers do differently: they leverage their time.

Time is incredibly democratic because it's the only resource that we all get the same amount of. What the world's smartest people do differently is pack maximum results into minimum investments of time. That's what distinguishes the top performers. They know the value of their time.

And that's what OsteoStrong delivers - the fastest results with the minimum amount of exercise and maximum amount of growth.

Yet this technology is not exclusive to the Lebron James and pro athletes of the world. What is so beautiful about what they've created is that it's for just about anyone at any level, from Olympic athletes to people suffering with chronic pain, to our elderly brothers and sisters.

You're about to unleash the kind of fitness, agility, strength and energy you really want. And the best part is, you'll have the easiest shortcut to reach your peak performance faster and pain-free.

Who wouldn't like a higher level of physical freedom? Who wouldn't love to feel powerful and strong with each step? Think of what you could accomplish if you felt strong and powerful. How would it change the way you show up in your life?

The better you feel, the more energy you'll have to produce amazing results in all the other areas of your life. The simple truth is that if you don't master your health, those other areas of life - your business, your relationships, your finances - probably won't live up to your ultimate vision. Because if you're lacking energy and vitality, you're lacking a strong foundation.

There's a great quote you've probably heard before: "A healthy person has a thousand wishes, a sick person only one." *Health is your ultimate wealth.*

I want you to know that I'm speaking to you as a brother. I'm speaking to you from my own experience of how my health has changed, and how I know your strength, vitality and health can be unleashed.

I feel incredibly blessed to share this gift with you because I know that these tools can transform your body like they have mine. I know that you can live your life with ultimate impact and passion. The possibilities are endless. Giving yourself this foundation of strength will enable you to be more, live more and give more. It's the ultimate gift you can give yourself.

So I honor you, and I welcome you to the next life-changing level of physical strength, vitality, and freedom.

PREFACE

John Jaquish, PhD

Creating a super-human version of yourself, regardless of your age or current physical condition, is no longer a daunting or unachievable goal. Gone are the days of "no pain, no gain."

Recent discoveries in health and medical science now allow us to maximize our body's potential - often more efficiently than with traditional diet and exercise techniques. The passion for optimizing health and performance of many dedicated health and wellness thought leaders and researchers has unlocked many new tools and strategies that were unknown to science only a few decades ago.

Have you ever wanted a more powerful body?

Imagine yourself with an unbreakable foundation of bones, muscles, ligaments, and tendons, free from pain, and boosted in energy, health, and healing by cutting-edge discoveries about how our bodies work. Imagine maximizing your freedom to experience life on your terms.

This may be easy to imagine. But too often, the road to achieving this level of health seems like a utopian fantasy. The effort, time commitment, and physical pain that is necessary to make these transformations real seems impossible.

If making this utopia a reality doesn't interest you, you can put this book down now. But if you'd like to explore a faster, easier path to stronger bones, stronger muscles, better health, and more energy - this is the book for you.

This isn't like other health and fitness books. We're not going to discuss traditional weight training routines, fad diets, or the usual basic lecture about "exercise and eating right."

Instead, we're going to introduce you to cutting-edge technologies and scientific discoveries which will empower you to gain health, strength, and longevity faster and more easily than you ever imagined.

What's the secret? Science. We're not going to skimp on the science in this book. We *will* make it fun to read and easy to understand, but you're going to come out of this understanding exactly *why* these technologies work, and why many other methods don't.

In some places we'll cite scholarly articles in case you *really* want to know what methods were used to obtain these findings, or which cellular signaling cascade is responsible for these astonishing effects.

We'll discuss the cellular biology and clinical evidence underlying each of these "hacks," and explain why they work so much better than other approaches to the same problems. We'll discuss pieces of technology you've probably never heard of that are available to you right now.

From eliminating and preventing serious diseases like osteoporosis and diabetes to "hacking" your body for optimal human performance, the doctors, scientists and inventors in this book have developed a new generation of hacks that provide superior health, strength, and wellness while minimizing the time, energy, and effort required to get them.

This is a book for sick people, healthy people, high-performance athletes, the elderly, and young people. We all share the same human biology - and that biology can be used by anyone for improved health and fitness. Many of the technologies we'll discuss here are the most effective modalities available on the market for age-related diseases such as osteoporosis, osteoarthritis, and back pain.

Perhaps unsurprisingly, the same technologies that can stimulate the body to trigger massive strength gains and healing in cases of disease and injury can *also* be used by healthy people to maximize muscle growth, metabolism, mood, energy levels, and general health.

The best news of all is this: these techniques are easy, and can massively affect physical performance and health for just about anyone, regardless of age or present level of physical fitness. Most of these technologies don't even require massive time commitments to pursue.

This book isn't about training *more* or adhering to a strictly regimented diet.

It's about training *smarter* by using new technologies to get better results with a fraction of the time and energy required for traditional methods.

Hard work is important to achieving any goal. Of course it is. But when it comes to health and fitness, working hard on the wrong approach can be useless, or even dangerous.

How many of you know someone who sustained an injury because they were trying to strengthen their bodies, but went about it in the wrong way? How many of you know someone who tried a diet craze or health fad, only to make their overall health *worse?*

And, more importantly, how many of you know someone who got *better* results than they expected from a new exercise or health routine? How many of you have heard someone say "I can't believe how easy that was" about gaining health or strength?

I'm guessing you know a lot fewer people in that second category. In part that's because we, as humans, are biologically designed to put minimal time and effort into everything. We have high standards for "quick" and "easy," which are rarely met by traditional diet and exercise techniques.

We have a built-in, ancient survival instinct built on these simple concepts: consume calories, conserve calories, and conserve energy. That's how we're built, and it makes sense when you think about what it must have taken to survive before the industrial revolution.

When I see someone who is carrying excess body fat, I know that their diet and exercise choices result from a biological hard-wired survival system designed to keep them alive through famine and hardship. But these same instincts actually work against humans in societies where food is abundant, and the days of hard physical work are long-gone for most.

That's not to say we can't enjoy an activity so much that we spend lots of time doing it. But generally, we have to manage our resources carefully. Often we can't *afford* to put lots of time and energy into pursuing a goal beyond basic survival. This is true for us today because of the busy modern world - it was true for our ancestors tens of thousands of years ago because of their uncertain food supply.

There's also another important reason why we don't usually get *better* results than we expect. Many traditional exercise and training programs simply don't take full advantage of modern science and technology. Forms of exercise such as jogging, weight-lifting, and sports have been around for thousands of years.

Until recently, not many people had thought to apply modern technology to re-invent strength training entirely based on modern understandings of how the body is wired to make stronger muscles and bones much more effectively.

We'll talk about more than just exercise and strength in this book.

We'll also talk about electromagnetic fields, which can be used to improve a huge variety of illnesses, injuries, and chronic conditions such as depression by enhancing the function of many important molecules in our body. While your doctor's office may not have a Pulsed Electromagnetic Field device yet, we'll discuss the most reliable manufacturers of over-the-counter versions and facilities where you can use them for a fraction of the cost of purchasing one for your home.

Lastly, we'll talk about red light therapy devices, which have been shown to have startling effects on health and healing thanks to a previously unknown biochemical pathway in the human mitochondria. We'll meet the professional athletes, cosmetologists, and self development experts who use these devices, and see how you can procure their benefits for yourself.

Specific technologies and scientific discoveries we'll cover include:

- OsteoStrong's osteogenic loading devices. Put simply, these are devices that trigger massive bone and muscle growth by exerting many times your normal body weight upon your body. Sounds scary, right? But osteogenic loading devices are actually safer than traditional exercise for many, and yield superior results.

  We'll discuss why and how these devices work, and where you can find facilities to take advantage of them.

- Electromagnetic energy, and how it affects your health. Pulsed Electromagnetic Fields (PEMF) are one cutting-edge technology used in many hospitals and clinics to promote healing and even fight cancers.

  You might ask how a single treatment could have so many different applications. We'll cover how different types of electromagnetic fields affect your body - for better or worse - and how they can stimulate blood flow, healing action, and even brain activity.

  We'll also discuss the difference between healing currents and the harmful-to-useless "electrosmog" produced by many household electronic devices.

- Red light therapy devices, which use cutting-edge discoveries about our biochemistry to deliver healing, youth, and vitality.

  You'll learn which wavelengths of light to look for in your own red light therapy device, how to properly measure your device's power, and more.

The objective of this book is to not just point out different "things" that you can do for your health. The list of techniques that can be used to improve health and fitness is nearly endless. But here, we'll offer those that have performed best in our analyses of cost of use, time investment, and power.

This is a critical value, as many "biohacks" do work - but may be extremely costly and offer comparatively little benefit. It can be difficult to tell which are the best investments, among the large numbers of claims about techniques or procedures that are "good for your health."

For example, there is a biohacking device that has become popular in the last few years. It combines cold water therapy and vascular occlusion (blood pressure cuffs which tighten to reduce blood flow to your limbs).

Cold water, or cold in general, tends to distract people from the intensity of an exercise, making it feel more tolerable. It also increases the number of calories burned, as your body must burn more calories simply to stay warm.

Restriction of blood flow using vascular occlusion has additional benefits: it increases the body's production of growth hormone (GH)/IGF-1 by an average of 15%. Many people are interested in increasing their body's natural release of GH/IGF hormones as they have powerful anti-aging effects, and their presence in the body normally decreases as a person ages.

But the device that offers these dual benefits is complex, computer-operated, and is almost the size of a small automobile. It costs nearly $50,000 dollars.

By comparison, scientists have discovered that five minutes spent doing squats on a vibrating platform increased IGF-1 by an average of *30%* - a much greater gain for a much, much smaller expenditure of time, energy, and money.

Improving the amount of gain you get for the time and energy you put in is my passion. In 2016, for example, I performed a meta-analysis looking at the results of 23 different studies and peer-reviewed published data sets that examined changes to levels of growth hormone with different types of exercise.

Based on this analysis, I identified a type of exercise that increased growth hormone by 400% - 2600% - a much greater gain than either of the techniques discussed above!

So whether you're seeking to improve a dangerous health condition, or looking to get the body of your dreams, read on and see how recent discoveries in science show the way to improved muscle and bone health, improved metabolism, and more.

INTRODUCTION

Kyle Zagrodzky

The book you are about to read is the product of many authors. It's primarily a labor of love on the part of biomedical engineer John Jaquish, PhD and myself.

In our passion for maximizing the physical health of ourselves and others, we've reached out to other wellness professionals who are on the cutting-edge of biological self-development, including people on the cutting-edge of Red Light Therapy and Pulsed Electromagnetic Field (PEMF, also known as high-tech "earthing" or "grounding") technology, which has been shown by clinical research to be effective for a vast array of health conditions.

This might sound like a dizzying variety of expertise to bring together in one book. But our health is a whole-body system: from the principles of cellular function to the biomechanics of movement and strength, optimizing health, fitness, and human ability is a multidisciplinary effort.

Our aim is to put together the book that will help you most. We have chosen not to review all things biohacking, but have instead focused on a narrow range biohacks which provide a far-reaching effect for a minimal input of effort. This means that implementing most or all of the different biohacks contained within this book should be easy, fun, and cost-effective.

These biohacks aren't just meant for athletes: they will be at least as useful to those suffering from low bone density, diabetes, obesity, and other common health concerns which can make traditional exercise difficult.

You may wonder why you haven't heard about some of these hacks before. The reason is simple: many people on the cutting-edge of scientific research are not entrepreneurs, or simply do not have the capital backing to make their findings widely available to the public.

Dr. Jaquish and I are fortunate to share a powerful combination of these traits. In addition to valuing medical science and data collection, we also have the entrepreneurial skills to make our findings available outside of the setting of medical facilities, or the pages of clinical research studies.

The best example I could find of a key factor that turns a new discovery into a lifestyle revolution can be found in the story of Asa Candler, the founder of Coca Cola.

In the mid 1800's Candler purchased the recipe for Coca Cola, an iron kettle, and wooden paddle from the doctor who came up with the formulation. The doctor had used his own expertise to develop the product, but had not managed to make it highly marketable or fully explain how delicious it was to the general public.

Candler invested his entire life savings of $500 - close to $16,000 in today's money - in buying the recipe and the equipment to make it. The difference between the doctor who had come up with the formula and Mr. Candler was, in essence, imagination.

Asa Candler saw the potential of what could be if this product were widely marketed, where the doctor could not. The product's discoverer had been content to use the recipe on a small scale, serving it only to his patients, family, and friends. And we know the rest of the story.

Coca Cola ushered in a new industry. This product alone has employed hundreds of thousands of people around the world, making billions of dollars, funding institutions, real estate projects, stadiums, etc.. And all of that was made possible, not by the man who discovered the formula, but by the man who had the insight to market it to the masses. I would say that was quite a good return on an investment of $500.

We like to make sure that inventors are credited for their work, and we've included the writings of several inventors - including Dr. Jaquish - here. But we also recognize that persistence and desire make the difference between an invention that can help a small number of people and an invention that can change the world.

It is my belief that we are all constantly surrounded by opportunities. We only need the imagination to see them, and an abundance of resourcefulness to transform them into reality.

Many people have the imagination to see the potentials of what could be, but two other ingredients are required to bring the imagination to life: desire and persistence.

In my experience, imagination is the most abundant of these three characteristics of success. Less common is another ingredient: desire. Rarest of all is the Holy Grail of success: persistence.

As my friend and business partner, Tony Robbins has often said:

"Execution wins over intelligence almost every time."

I've taken the liberty to create a formula for execution:

Imagination + Desire + Persistence = Execution.

Dr. Jaquish is a rare breed with the acute imagination to see in clinical research the potential others have missed. Together, our combination of skills, imagination, desire and persistence have manifested a new family of biohacks into reality.

What is being created by us and other biohackers using cutting-edge science is the dawn of a new era of human capability. An era where science is combined with imagination to yield incredible gains for the average person.

I am not a researcher and I do not hold a PhD. I do, however, have an intense imagination and an almost obsessive need to create plans and execute my ideas.

Before I met Dr. Jaquish, I had turned this drive into a series of fitness franchises which offered traditional health and fitness equipment to the public. Since meeting him, my vision of what a fitness franchise can be has been revolutionized by his totally unique equipment designs, and the unprecedented benefits that come with them.

Don't worry - this isn't a sales book. We will recommend the best products we know of to help you reach goals like strong and healthy bones, rapid strength gains, optimal health and healing, healthy mood and sleep. But our main purpose is to discuss the science underlying each of these biohacks so that you will have a better understanding of how and why they work.

From the cellular biology of muscle strength to the biochemistry of health and healing, here you'll learn the essentials you need to biohack your body to its fullest potential regardless of your health state, and with less effort than ever before.

At my core, I am driven by two questions. The first question I always ask myself is:

How can this be better?

I ask this question almost constantly, even if the process I'm considering has nothing to do with me, my family or my business. The urge to make things the best that they can be seems innate.

The second question I ask is this:

What drives people to take action?

Most of the problems in our world today - be they personal

health problems or global crises - stem simply from lack of action. In this scientific era, we *know* how to solve nearly every problem we face quickly and effectively. But we often don't put that knowledge into practice in our daily lives. Why?

That is the question I ask daily. I study both helpful and harmful actions. I study the things people spend money, time, and energy on - for better or worse.

When it comes to inventions and new knowledge, the most powerful inventions are only as effective as the people who take action to use them. Only when new knowledge is widely understood and integrated into daily life can it truly change the world.

That's what this book is all about. Here we'll share some of the latest discoveries and inventions in health and fitness with you. You might be amazed to discover what scientists know - but have largely failed to communicate to the public.

In 1997, my wife and I owned nine Curves fitness franchises. A few years later, we would be awarded franchise owners of the year. This was before we met any of these inventors or biohackers, when we felt our mission in life was to encourage people to use traditional gym equipment to stay healthy and strong. Little did we know how much untapped potential for enhanced health and fitness lay in relatively unknown technologies.

Fortunately, we were able to learn about cutting-edge biohacks in the years to come. This happened because I have always been motivated by two things: first, a desire to help people become a better version of themselves. Second: seeing how technology can help them achieve greater results, faster.

I wasn't interested in creating new technology, but I was interested in technology as a tool that could be leveraged to make better use of time. Any successful business owner will tell you that time - not money - is our greatest asset, and that success is dictated by how wisely a person uses their time.

After all, we can make or lose money - but no amount of wealth can add extra hours to the day, or extra years to your life (unless you use wealth to support longevity-expanding lifestyle choices like those we'll talk about here).

In 1997, I started a software company whose purpose was to alleviate the mundane and repetitive work associated with running our Curves centers. I wanted the software to accomplish two objectives: to save time, and to create better data collection and better visibility for the metrics needed to run our centers.

My effort to constantly improve my franchise's offerings were directed by a philosophy I learned in my Curves training that has always stayed with me:

"The best type of exercise for someone is the one they'll do."

The health and fitness industry has seen massive innovations in both technological capabilities and customer experience over the past two decades. But through it all, the industry is constantly trying to achieve one overriding objective: to provide a fitness service that people will actually use.

All that really matters at the end of the day is whether people show up and exercise. You might have the most miraculous equipment in the world, but if no one uses it, you haven't had much of an impact.

Yet despite all of the changes and advancements in recent decades, the percentage of people in the United States that both have a gym membership and actually use it regularly floats around 4%. That's not much of a change from the situation we had decades ago.

With that knowledge, I became more and more fascinated by human nature as it relates to fitness. After all, today almost everyone knows the benefits of traditional exercise, from longer lifespan to better health and an improved emotional state. But 96% of people in our society don't act on this knowledge.

Why not?

Every year, we see hundreds of thousands of people commit to a gym membership in an effort to get healthier. Their intentions are good and their commitment is sincere, but each year we see the same pattern time and again. Many join, and almost as many quit in a few months or less despite having made the resolution to better their health and live longer.

In recent decades, the fitness industry has seen massive strides in perfecting the available methods and systems of fitness, as well as mastering the art of customer service. But the one constant is that most people can't stick with it.

With my built-in driving questions, "How can this be better?" and "What causes people to take action?" I have obsessed over what needs to change for people to stay with it.

I have searched in earnest to understand the components of human nature that cause us to avoid the very thing (exercise) that has mountains of evidence supporting the certainty that it will help us all live better lives.

In the early nineties, I and many others purchased Tony Robbins' self-development course, "Personal Power." What was contained on those tapes forever changed the course of my life.

One of the many things I have never forgotten is that human beings, at their core, are pleasure-seekers and pain-avoiders. It's so simple, yet explains so much.

When it comes to fitness, I have concluded that there is a genetic reason people don't engage in fitness exercise on a large scale. It goes deeper than an emotional avoidance of the physical pain of exercise. The real reason is that we are beautifully designed to survive.

In order to survive, we must conserve calories. Calories are energy, and energy is life.

For the majority of Earth's history, and arguably for most places on Earth today, the availability of food has been uncertain. We must both conserve and store calories whenever possible; our biological foundation demands it.

Think about cheetahs, for instance. We don't see cheetahs running around the Serengeti at sixty miles an hour for the fun of it, or to keep their muscles strong. Quite the contrary: biologists have discovered that if a cheetah misses its prey after three chase attempts, there is a high likelihood it will die as a result of burning more calories running than it has stored as fat.

By the same token, the survival of any species has historically been very difficult. Just a few thousand years ago, high-energy foods such as domesticated wheat and potatoes, dairy products, sugar, and alcohol were not available to our ancestors.

Now that these foods are available, we crave them - so much so that diseases related to excess consumption of calories, carbohydrates, and sugars are now among the leading killers in the developed world. This, too, is a function of our beautiful design as calorie-conserving creatures.

Consuming and storing calories is a built-in genetic survival feature in every animal on the planet. So as I see people becoming more and more obese, I know that they are simply acting in the way that they are biologically wired to act.

Going against the grain of humanity's calorie-consuming and conserving nature is often a losing battle. In our minds, we know we must take care of ourselves. But this knowledge is often not sufficient to motivate us to overpower our instincts and produce lifestyle changes.

So how can we pursue good health by working *with* our genetic make-up, and not against it?

At their core, bio-hackers intuitively understand the answer to this question. A biohacker looks for ways to hack human biology to achieve their desired results, with the smallest expenditure of time and energy (calories) possible. This means they face little or no resistance from their own deepest instincts when implementing these biohacks.

Biohacking is here to stay, and thank God for that. It is my belief that only this kind of mindset will save us from spiraling healthcare costs as a result of progressively less healthy lifestyles.

This book will focus on an array of specific modern-day biohacks that you will actually feel tempted to do, because they are easy and even fun. We will discuss the science behind each of them, and ultimately, how you can access them yourself.

This will likely not be the last edition of this book. True biohackers like Dr. Jaquish, Dave Asprey, Ben Greenfield, and Tim Ferris live in constant pursuit of the next best biohack.

John and I will work to present these methods as they manifest themselves into reality in future editions of this book, and in future blogs and podcasts.

Your engagement in bettering your physical health for increased happiness, health, and freedom is our ultimate goal.

We hope that you will read, learn, implement, and share what you find in these pages.

Biohacking is an idea whose time has come.

CHAPTER 1

Unbreakable Bones
John Jaquish, PhD

THIS CHAPTER IS for the old and the young. It's for people suffering from osteoporosis, and for high-performance athletes.

That's true of *all* the chapters in this book, but it's especially true of this one. What we discuss here will be foundational for all the other biohacks contained within this book.

If our skeletal system is not in order, our muscles, organ systems, and energy levels can't be. So whether you're seeking to recover from frail health or seeking to push your athletic game to the next level, read on as we discuss the one thing that all of us have in common: our skeletal systems.

If you put a Formula 1 engine into an economy car, what would happen? Car buffs know the answer to this question: the powerful engine would completely destroy the car.

That's because an everyday passenger car is not made to handle the powerful forces produced by a Formula 1 engine. The car's frame, its wheels and axel, its brakes and steering - all would shatter across the pavement if the auto equivalent of a jet engine were suddenly strapped onboard.

Did you know that the same principle applies to our own bodies?

Many athletes are puzzled by why they hit a plateau in muscle or strength, or why they seem to stop gaining strength even though they continue to train. There's one common, but relatively unknown reason for this: our bodies won't let our muscles exert forces powerful enough to break our bones.

It's a good thing we have this failsafe built in! Imagine being able to make a fist tight enough to break your own fingers, or being able to run so fast that your ankle shattered from the force. That would have spelled instant death for an ancient human running from a lion, so the body put checks and balances in place.

When our muscles contract so hard they're at risk of deforming our bones, our central nervous system actually sends inhibitory signals to tell our nerves to stop the muscle from exerting any more force. This is called neural inhibition, and it's there to protect you.

In other words, if you try to grow your muscle strength, but your skeletal frame isn't powerful enough to handle these forces, you will not get strength benefits from your exercise. Your body will prevent the muscle from doing more than your bones can handle, and your apparent strength gain will stop.

This applies to osteoporosis and physical therapy patients just as much as it applies to professional athletes and bodybuilders. Whatever muscle strength you achieve must be matched by bone strength, if you want to continue seeing strength gains.

Unfortunately, until recently it was believed that bone growth largely stopped after adolescence. Conventional wisdom said that exercise later in life could prevent bone loss, but could not build new bone where there had been none before.

In other words, those seeking to gain radical muscle strength later in life were out of luck. They had a limiting factor built into their very bones.

In recent years, however, findings across several fields of science have shown that this conventional picture just isn't true. We now know that radical gains in bone mass density - a measure of the strength of bones - can be experienced at any age, if the proper technologies are used to "tell" our bodies to make new bone safely.

It may be true that walking or jogging won't build new bone later in life, but what if we found a safe and hyper-effective way to replicate the conditions experienced by the athletes who develop the strongest bones of all: professional gymnasts?

This chapter is the story of OsteoStrong. It's the story of how I developed a device to replicate - and even exceed - the bone-generating signals experienced by the highest-performance athletes, and packed that benefit into a safe, easy, low-impact activity that can be performed for a few minutes per week in a gym or clinic for staggering results.

Sound too good to be true? Here we'll discuss the peer-reviewed research that led me to this design, and the bone strength gains we've seen in those who use it.

The Mother of Invention

My journey into biohacking began in a surprising way. I was neither a pro-athlete nor a bone density patient. Instead, I was a student - with a very big problem to solve.

I came home to my parents' house on a Sunday afternoon like so many students, eager to eat the largest meal possible and get my laundry done.

I walked through the door of my parents' home with food on my mind. But when I saw the look on my mother's face, I immediately lost my appetite. She looked upset. Bleak. Like she'd just received terrible news.

What could have upset her so badly?

My mother told me she had been to see her physician on Friday. She had undergone a DXA scan (a bone density measurement taken using a dual x-ray device) just a few weeks before my visit, and had gotten her results just before I arrived.

Her physician told her that she was diagnosed with osteoporosis - a loss of bone density that put her at risk for mobility problems, and for injuries that could become life-threatening as she got older.

Now, my mother had a history of unnecessarily worrying about all kinds of things. My father even had to hide a medical dictionary we had in the library of our house that she had started reading for fun. Everything she read about in that medical dictionary, she imagined she had. From malaria, all the way down to diseases that have not been seen in North America for 50+ years.

However, it soon became clear that this was different. She had been diagnosed by a doctor, using state-of-the-art imaging tests. And as a woman in her early 60s, she was in a high-risk group for osteoporosis.

I asked to see her DXA scan, and told her I was going to learn more about this. I'd never been one to take bad news lying down, and if there was a way to save my mother from these risks, I was going to find it.

At the time, I was studying for a business degree. This was my dad's idea. Though I'd always had a passion for biology and an interest in the human body, my dad had informed me that a business degree was the only college degree he'd pay for.

I later found out that he'd told my mother that "science comes so easily to the kid," and that if I learned business as well, I'd be the master of my own destiny. He turned out to be right - but probably not in the way he expected.

Although I was a business student with no intention of becoming a doctor at the time, I knew more than most about the human body. And my mother's case gave me all the more reason to study it. If she had a disease that would put her at risk of increased injury, I wanted to know everything about it.

I went to the university library to read books on radiology, and learn how to interpret some of the metrics on the scan. I learned that her bone density was right at the osteoporosis diagnosis level. This means a "T score" of lower than -2.5, which was exactly where she was.

She had osteoporosis, but just barely. Medical expectations predicted that it would inevitably get worse as she got older, as most people lose more and more bone density with age, and almost no one had been observed to build *more* bone density.

But I wondered why that was. Could anything be done to reverse her condition, instead of allowing it to get worse?

Conventional wisdom at the time said "no." Many believed that exercise and diet could prevent osteoporosis early in life, but could not reverse it once it had begun. For that reason, people were - and still are - encouraged to walk, run, and eat nutrient-rich diets to build bone density early in childhood and young adulthood. That would build strong, healthy bones at the time when the human body was growing most - so that when bone loss started later, it would be less of a problem.

While this is still excellent advice for young people, it didn't help my mother. Conventional wisdom said that, with age, the body stopped producing new bone. Once bone density was lost, it was thought that there was nothing that could be done to grow or replace it.

There were pharmaceutical options to slow down bone loss, which should reduce the risk of injury. But like all pharmaceuticals, they had side effects on other organ systems. I knew my mother did not want to take medications, and I could understand why. So I told her to be patient, as I was going to keep reading about what else could be done.

The idea that the body stopped producing new bone entirely with age seemed intuitively wrong to me. We don't stop healing broken bones after the age of twenty, after all, so our bone-building function could not be completely dormant.

Was there a way to safely trigger the same repair function throughout the body, to prevent injury instead of healing it? It seemed as though there should be.

I soon discovered that osteoporosis happens because our bodies only make what they think we need. Bone, muscle, and other tissues are lost if we don't use them.

This is a brilliant attempt by our bodies to conserve resources. Since humans originally existed in an environment of scarcity, our bodies assume it's better to conserve resources than to put calories and protein and minerals into building bones and muscles that we aren't using.

If we're not exerting force on our bones and muscles on a regular basis, our body's logic goes, we must not need them. And it's better to cut back than to spend nutrients and calories maintaining something that isn't vital to our daily life.

The most extreme example of this is found in astronauts who spend time in space. In space, there's no pull of gravity for them to push against. This means their bones and muscles - even their heart muscles! - don't need to work as hard.

As a result, the body decides that the astronaut doesn't "need" new bone and muscle cells, and simply stops replacing these cells when they age and die.

With no gravity to fight against, astronauts lose huge amounts of bone and muscle density even though they do resistance exercises which simulate the pull of gravity for a minimum of two hours per day. This two-hour-per-day exercise minimum is NASA's effort to convince their astronauts' bodies that they really *do* need bone and muscle tissues - so they will still be able to walk and pump blood to their brains against the force of gravity when they arrive back on Earth.

Then I discovered the opposite end of the spectrum in, of all places, the gymnastics world.

I discovered that gymnasts had the highest bone density of any group of people studied by scientists. I also discovered that clinical studies had found that "high impact" exercise - exercises such as jumping jacks and running, which cause the body to "impact" the ground after being airborne - were positively correlated with high bone density.

That made good sense. Gymnastics is, after all, the ultimate high-impact sport. We've all seen the Olympic gymnasts who jump high into the air and even do flips, before catching themselves gracefully on stunningly strong arms and legs.

What we can't see from the sidelines is the amount of force that puts on their bones.

When the body impacts the ground at a high velocity, it briefly experiences far more G-force than normal Earth gravity. In the instant when they hit the ground, gymnasts' bodies can experience forces more than ten times stronger than those we experience in the course of normal walking or running.

In my research, a pattern was beginning to emerge. Lack of weight on the bones led to rapid, alarming deterioration; putting additional weight on our bones with the minor impacts of running or jumping jacks, or the major ones of gymnastics, seemed to increase bone density.

It was as though these high-impact activities "told" our bodies we needed to grow new bone to withstand these strong forces. And the more intense the impact, the more intense the effect on bone growth seemed to be.

You might ask how this is possible. After all, for many years scientists believed that our bodies could only grow in the ways they were genetically programmed to grow, and that a person's lifestyle couldn't substantially alter their growth patterns or physical abilities.

It has always been somewhat obvious that this was wrong. Exercise has always increased muscle strength, and people living in extreme environments have always developed different abilities from others. But scientists did not know how this worked until the last few decades, when they discovered dozens of unseen "chemical messengers" within our bodies.

These messengers are chemicals that bind to receptors on a cell, and change the way that cell operates. They may change gene expression, metabolism, or cause the cell to send out other messengers of its own throughout the body.

Through this ingenious system, our bodies can trigger massive changes such as puberty, wound healing, and fight-or-flight responses in response to signals from inside and outside our own bodies.

It turns out that some of these signals tell our bodies to create new bone. But these signals are only released - and this is crucial - when our bones experience forces strong enough to bend our bones. We'll look at the peer-reviewed research showing this effect from high-impact exercise later in this chapter.

When our bones experience so much force that they can't hold their shape anymore, our body receives the message that our bones aren't dense enough to do their jobs.

We don't have *enough* bone to cope with our current circumstances. Therefore, we need to make more. Chemical messengers are released, and bone-creating cells called "osteoblasts" go to work laying down the matrix of tissue that will become new bone.

This discovery that bone density could be gained under extreme impact conditions still left me with a problem.

High-impact exercises like running and gymnastics were obviously not a great choice for people with osteoporosis. The average gymnast retires by the age of nineteen due to injuries; having an older person who is already unusually prone to injury due to osteoporosis try the same training routines wouldn't be safe.

So, what could be done? Was there a way to get the benefits of high-impact exercise without the risks?

When our bones experience forces so extreme that they realize they must become stronger, the application of these high forces is called "osteogenic loading." The "osteo" means "bone," and the "genic" is for "generating." The loading refers to the amount of force, or load, that we put on our bones.

"Osteogenic loading" is literally "bone-generating force."

As I studied the way doctors and scientists talked about bone growth and exercise, I realized that wasn't really the *impact* that was important. It was the *load* placed on our bones. And under normal circumstances, creating high-force impacts of the body on the ground by jumping high into the air was the only way to increase this load.

But what if there was another way to do it, using forces beyond the force of gravity to load weight onto our bones?

Normally, we experience about 1G of loading on our bones - the weight of our bodies under Earth's gravity. Astronauts in space experience 0G, or zero osteogenic load, while runners experience slightly more than 1G when their feet impact the ground, and gymnasts can experience more than 10Gs when landing from a jump.

These rapid changes in force on the body caused serious injuries in most high-impact athletes, and they definitely weren't right for patients like my mom who had osteoporosis.

But could there be a way to increase the amount of osteogenic loading our bones experience in a slow, controlled fashion, without the sudden, uncontrolled changes in force that injured so many gymnasts?

In theory, it could be done. By building a machine that loaded the body with artificial weight - but slowly, in a controlled and predictable fashion - it should be possible to replicate the osteogenic loading of high-impact sports, without the risk of injury.

I began to study the impact positions used by gymnasts to create their stunningly strong bones.

What angles were their legs and bodies at when they hit the ground? What positions allowed that force to be distributed throughout their skeletal systems, resulting in reduced risk of injury and greater bone density across the body?

How could I replicate that in a stable, stationary setup that would safely and gradually load weight onto the body's most important bones?

It soon became clear that to make my theory a reality, I'd need robotics, computer software, and a huge amount of steel.

By this point, a few years had passed while I conducted my research into how to help people like my mother with osteoporosis. I was now in graduate school, and working in software sales to help pay the bills.

This was tremendously helpful: to design a device optimized for osteogenic loading and capture data to make sure it was really working, I would need to determine how to capture and manage a lot of data. I would also need the help of a brilliant mechanical engineer.

Fortunately, I happened to know one. The problem was, it would be very difficult to get him involved.

Why? Because he was my father.

Fathers want to believe in their kids, but they also remember every mistake you ever made as a kid. They remember every window you broke, every time you tracked mud through the house, and every dent on the car that somehow appeared when you were out late with your friends.

This can have an effect on our fathers' perceptions of our foresight, or lack thereof. At some level, they're always looking for the flaw in your crazy idea and expecting it to end like the time you jumped out of that tree with wings made from bedsheets strapped to your back.

My father was no exception.

As I sat down with him and explained how I believed I could reverse mom's bone loss with a medical device I had conceptualized, he was exceedingly skeptical.

If this worked, he asked, why hadn't it been done before? Maybe the other scientists who figured this out didn't know any mechanical engineers, I suggested hopefully. Then I presented him with the peer-reviewed data that clearly showed bone growth with high-impact exercise.

Why couldn't we do this for mom? If it worked for these high-performance athletes - couldn't we at least try a version that might work for her?

I knew this would be the toughest sale I was ever going to have to make.

I ended up drawing on a cocktail napkin to illustrate how we could create a metal structure that could be customized to the individual biomechanics of different patients. A series of chains, gears, and variable pressure devices could be adjusted for height, weight, and different levels of bone and muscle strength.

With a platform like this, there was no reason we couldn't deliver several body weights of force - safely, and for much longer periods of time than the microsecond impacts experienced by gymnasts.

My father finally agreed to do the engineering CAD work to design the prototype, and then the final device. I promised to recruit a software engineer to create a program that would run the machine properly - and gather data about its effectiveness.

The software component proved to be more complicated than I'd anticipated. The software engineers I recruited told me it would have to include:

- Software that would encourage slow and controlled movements for safety, even as users emulated high-impact forces like those experienced by gymnasts.

- A system that was cloud-based, meaning all data was stored securely on the Internet. This would make it easy to compare and analyze the data from all sources when multiple devices were being used in the future.

- Integration of load-measuring hardware and robotics so that all experiences on the system would be accurate and repeatable.

It's hard to put innovation on a timeline. When you're creating something that has never existed, there are always unexpected challenges. This is especially true when taking a prototype designed in some guy's garage to market as a sleek, streamlined commercial device.

The first prototypes of the device were not going to win any beauty contests. They were made of big wooden blocks, chains, load sensors, computer screens, and seat pads made out of old beach towels wrapped in duct tape. I couldn't hire a factory to build something when I knew it would need improvements after I'd collected data, so many components of the first device were home-made, cobbled together out of existing parts.

This was the second-hardest sale I had to make in my life. I had to convince my 60-something mother to use an exercise machine that looked like a torture device.

I promised her that I believed this could reverse her trend of bone loss, and reduce her risk of injury in the future. I showed her the data, just as I had shown my father.

At the time I believed that simply stopping the degradation would be a success, since an average postmenopausal female loses between 1.5 and 2.5% of her bone mass per year. Gains in bone density, while theoretically possible, were still a long-shot dream for me.

The device was controlled via chains. The user (my mother, in this case) could adjust them to get into the four positions that I had identified as the impact absorption positions that would distribute the machine's force across all of her load bearing bones

There was a movement which placed osteogenic loading on the arms, from the hands to the upper rib cage. There was a movement for the legs all the way to the hip joint, a movement for the core, and lastly one for the neck and spine.

With these four positions, I hoped we'd isolate all of the bone groups which were in danger of injury from everyday activities during aging. The descendants of these positions, refined over the course of years of trial, error, and engineering, can still be seen in today's OsteoStrong devices.

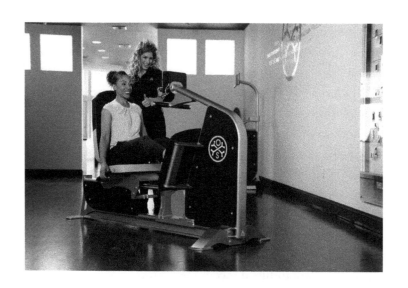

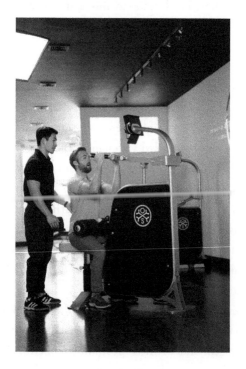

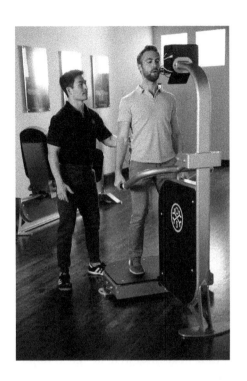

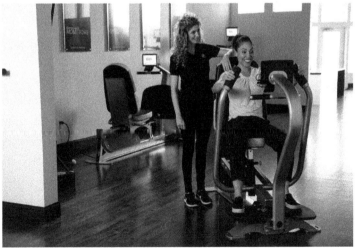

With reluctance, my mother began to use the first primitive version of this device. And then the next one, after I made some improvements for comfort.

Even though she didn't like the look of it, she quickly learned that she could feel the difference the device was making. Each time she used it, the force she could safely exert on her bones during the next session increased.

I call the amount of loading a user's bones can safely handle "functional bone performance." This measures not just the strength of one individual bone, but the entire musculoskeletal system working together, to yield a real-world estimate of how prepared a user's body is to handle accidental or intentional impact force.

Whether it's deadlifting weights or missing a stair, we all deal with sudden, powerful forces on our bodies at one time or another. These are the forces that can cause life-threatening injuries for osteoporosis patients - and these are the forces that my "Impact Emulation" machines were designed to prepare the body to handle safely.

When my mother used the loading device, she didn't just put load onto her bones. She also increased the load on her tendons, ligaments, cartilage, and muscle tissue.

Our software readouts told us that the machine was working, in the sense of delivering the promised forces on my mother's musculoskeletal system. But there was one important measurement we still need to learn if the osteogenic loading theory was working. Only time - and bone scans - would tell if her bone density loss had slowed or stopped since she began using the device.

Even before those results were observed, I had a strong feeling that my invention was going to change millions of lives. I watched my previously inactive mother seem to grow stronger, more coordinated, and more confident in her body's abilities.

As she became more accustomed to making a range of movements in a controlled setting, she also seemed to become more confident in her ability to handle new tasks and activities in everyday life. It was so simple, yet made so much sense.

We went through several iterations of the machine as I took measurements based on my mother's use, adjusted, and refined.

After 18 months of my mother using the devices, we got her first Post-Impact Emulation bone density tests back. And we were thrilled!

My mother had not only completely reversed the bone loss - she had gained significant bone density, to the point where she no longer fit the diagnostic criteria for osteoporosis. She'd moved from diagnosis levels at the start of her history with the device (-2.54 T Score) to the bone density of an average female in her 30s (-0.3 T Score).

My mother was excited and relieved. The machine had effectively given her back thirty years of bone density. But we hardly had time to celebrate: now that we knew that this worked, I had to find a way to get the devices manufactured so that other patients could use them.

My father and I created one more iteration of the device: one that looked sleek, professional, and more like a piece of gym equipment than a torture device. I secured a deal with a manufacturer and started a clinic to house the new machines.

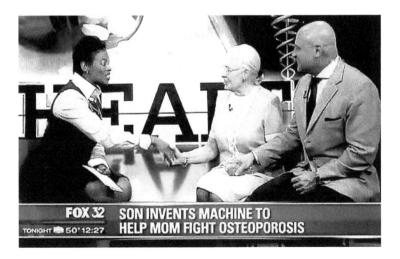

Then I began to help people use the devices.

Very quickly, my single location had hundreds of users. The elderly population embraced a machine that did not exhaust them or require high-impact activities like traditional gym equipment, and local athletes were always on the lookout for new ways to gain an edge on the competitive circuit.

I knew I needed to be able to demonstrate this effect in more users in order for this knowledge to spread, but at the time I still did not have my doctorate. I had approached this problem from the perspective of helping one person - my mother - and I had no real idea of how to scale it up, or bring my results to the scientific community.

Fortunately, the most amazing physician found my office and told me that she wanted to be a part of what I was doing. She had the knowledge I was missing: the knowledge of how to publish peer-reviewed research, and share my results with the scientific community.

Dr. Elenor Hynote was an internal medicine physician in Napa Valley, where my first clinic was located. She had heard about what I was doing, and believed that the concept jived with what she had been focusing on in her practice.

I didn't know it at the time, but she was the President of the American College for the Advancement of Medicine (ACAM).

This is an organization that puts physical medicine interventions first - meaning that they encourage pharmaceutical interventions only when all nutritional, physical therapy, and exercise options have been exhausted to treat any given dysfunction.

Dr. Hynote had been monitoring the bone density of several of her patients, who had been using my devices for eight months. After seeing significant improvements in their bone densities, she became interested in using our method herself. She had low bone density which was on track to develop into osteoporosis as she aged - and she knew that millions of other American women did, too.

She didn't just want to use our machines. She wanted to know every detail about the references I used to develop my theory, the engineering processes I'd used to create the machines, and the osteogenic loading effects which actually created new bone.

Through my discussions with Dr. Hynote, she emphasized that while I had created a strong case for the efficacy of this process, I did not yet have the ability to write and document my invention in an academic manner. Since I did not yet have any formal biology degree credentials, it would be almost impossible for my data to be published in peer-reviewed journals.

Dr. Hynote and I both knew that this publishing ability would give me the potential to inspire a movement in the mainstream medical community to prescribe and recommend the use of osteogenic loading for osteoporosis.

We also knew that this could change the face of the disease - which was a problem expected to reach epidemic proportions as the Baby Boomer population approached retirement age, and modern sedentary lifestyles cut down on natural osteogenic loading in the daily lives of young people.

Dr. Hynote offered to write letters of recommendation for me to several Biomedical Engineering Ph.D. programs. I could enter these programs with my own self-funded dissertation project - the study of the osteogenic loading process. Rushmore University responded positively to this request, and I began my work toward my degree.

After a few years of studying for my Ph.D. and running the osteogenic loading clinic, the data I had collected had shown compelling results in a large sample size. I published papers showing significant bone density gain in my device's users in the *Journal of Osteoporosis and Physical Activity* and *Osteoporosis International.*

I was also able to publish results showing improvement in A1c levels - an important indicator of the risk of organ damage from high blood sugar - in patients with diabetes and metabolic dysfunction after using Impact Emulation machines in the *Journal of Diabetes and Metabolism.*

Now, the scientific and medical communities were primed to understand that osteogenic loading really could be used to increase bone density, even in older people and patients with osteoporosis. We had even shown that this technology could help patients with other conditions, such as diabetes and metabolic dysfunction.

But I also needed something else: promotion of the technology from a marketing perspective.

It wasn't enough for doctors and scientists to know about this technology. The high price tag for installing the machine in clinics and the "only fix what's already broken" approach often applied in medical care meant that doctors alone wouldn't put the device into the hands of most of the people who could benefit from its effects.

My Impact Emulation design was safe, meaning it didn't require a prescription and could be pursued by anyone who lived near an osteogenic loading clinic or gym. This also allowed the device to be accessed affordably, since it didn't require close medical oversight or need to share space with expensive laboratory equipment.

That meant that the best way to spread its benefits was to create clinics and gyms equipped with these devices, and then tell the public about them.

The truth is, the expression "build a better mousetrap and the world will beat a path to your door" is profoundly wrong. If nobody knows you have a better mousetrap, nobody will show up. This can pose a challenge for inventors who are not marketing-savvy, or naturally good at self-promotion.

Fortunately, one of my first customers, whose health was massively improved by the device, knew the world-renowned Tony Robbins.

At this point, I had someone calling me every week and telling me that they were going to introduce me to some influential person (the U.S. Surgeon General, or the President, or whoever), and that they were going to help me get my technology "all over the world." I would just smile and nod, because most of these people were wishful thinkers who wanted to be involved with something big, but had no influence over these powerful people at all.

This guy who knew Tony Robbins however, was serious. I just didn't know it until one day, my phone rang.

The conversation went something like this:

"Hi there! My name is Tony, and I'd like to buy a set of your devices."

"Well, um…I only have prototypes, and right now they're costing me $300,000 per set to produce."

"Sure, no problem. I'll pay for a prototype set."

"…what was your name, again?"

When I delivered the prototype to Tony's house in Southern California, we had a great time discussing the unorthodox approach I had taken and the similarities to his own worldview. He'd learned that there is often a better, more direct solution to any given problem.

These solutions are often simple and easy: they just haven't been discovered yet because they're not obvious. He saw Impact Emulation as just such a breakthrough: something incredibly powerful that makes sense, but which isn't widely known because people are unlikely to stumble across it in the course of their daily lives.

He also told me that his primary work was not just inspiring people (though that was a huge part of what he did), but rather finding the most effective solutions for challenges that almost all people have. Inspiration goes much further, after all, when you apply it to the fastest and easiest techniques for success.

The challenges that Tony helped people tackle ranged from anxiety and confidence to health and wellness. So to him, Impact Emulation fit right in.

I was fascinated by what he was saying - and I couldn't wait to see how he could help me deliver the message of osteogenic loading via Impact Emulation.

After finishing my Ph.D., I took my dissertation and adapted it into a book that I could share with medical professionals. Those wishing to learn about the mechanisms of bone and muscle formation in far greater scientific detail and specificity may be interested in this book, which is available under the title <u>Osteogenic Loading: OsteoStrong Edition</u> through Amazon and other retailers.

In writing this book, I was lucky enough to have the help of Dr. Hynote and a neurologist, Dr. Raj Singh.

Dr. Singh was also published in peer-reviewed journals, and was extremely interested in the neurological activation that the devices could create. After all, these were whole-body machines: their unique forces and movements allowed for an unusual strengthening of nerve-muscle connections, as well as an unusual strengthening of bones and muscles.

With his help, we began to take my Impact Emulation devices to groups of medical doctors. I began encouraging them to install the devices in their practices, so that their patients could use them for a variety of bone, muscle, metabolic, and nerve-related applications.

While this endeavor was exciting, Tony and I both knew that this was not the big picture for osteogenic loading. Getting a set of devices into a physician's office meant that they would treat maybe twenty people who had acute health conditions with it and call it a smashing success.

But if I had to spend a few hours with a physician to only affect the lives of twenty people, this project would never be able to penetrate the broader population of billions who sought to enhance their health and fitness, or were facing bone density loss as they aged.

After expanding to one clinic at a time for a few years, I ended up at a physician's office in Memphis, Tennessee. They had an installation of my osteogenic loading devices, and I was there to give a lecture to a patient group about their benefits and proper use. Some potential referring physicians from the area had shown up as well, to hear about the new technology and see if what I was there to discuss could be right for their patients.

I noticed someone in the audience who was taking notes during the lecture, which was normal. But when I started to take the patients of the clinic through their first experiences with Impact Emulation, I noticed that he was timing me with his watch.

This was unique. Most people who listened to my presentations asked questions, but none of them had *timed* me before. I wondered what this unique spectator was thinking.

Fortunately, I was about to find out. He and I ended up having dinner at the home of a mutual friend who had invited him to my demonstration. I learned that his name was Kyle, and that he had been an owner of several fitness franchises and a large technology company.

As we talked, it became clear that he understood all of the challenges I faced in my work. And he knew exactly how to solve them.

He had a vision for osteogenic loading, just like I did. His business was to supply spaces where people could use machines that would help them to get fit. By creating a chain of facilities that specialized in osteogenic loading, he would be able to keep membership costs low and make devices available to thousands of people across a wide geographic area.

He had exactly what I needed: a way to make my devices available to the public.

This vision became OsteoStrong, and that man was OsteoStrong's founder, Kyle Zagrodzky. I knew as I shook his hand that night that my years of hard work were finally going to be accessible to the world.

If you're convinced by what you've read here, and feel you have a sufficient understanding of the mechanism of osteogenic loading, you can skip this next section and move on to our other biohacks. We're about to get very scientific - probably more scientific than you need to get if you're in a hurry.

But if you want to understand more of the mechanisms, evidence, and science behind osteogenic loading, read on. We're now embarking on a review of the medical science and peer-reviewed literature that has illuminated why - and how - osteogenic loading works.

The Science of Bone Growth

Bone density isn't a topic often discussed in sports performance circles, but it should be.

We're all called upon to exert maximal force at some time in our lives, be it trying to win a gold medal at the Olympics, or having to catch ourselves during a fall. This means that at some point, we will need all the power we have available to protect ourselves.

Osteogenic loading can deliver this by strengthening bone and removing a limitation on the growth of muscle strength by increasing the nervous system's activation of muscle, and by improving the force tolerance of the bone itself.

Previously, we have only seen this kind of musculoskeletal power in gymnasts and other high-performance athletes. These individuals are the only group who consistently absorbs these levels of force, and thereby have unbreakable levels of bone density and ability to exert and absorb force. They achieve this through years of grueling training, beginning in childhood and often ending with significant injuries during the teenage years.

Now, with osteogenic loading devices, we have the ability to safely bring these kinds of benefits to almost anyone at any age.

We have entered an uncharted era of human development.

The new technology described in this book enables osteogenic loading, or the growth of new bone mass through axial loading of the musculoskeletal system. This technology enables a new type of therapy and exercise in a simple, effective device that can be widely and safely prescribed for many populations.

In addition to improving strength and bone health, subjects using osteogenic loading have greatly increased muscular force production, which improves balance and reduces the risk of falls and injuries in elderly populations. The principles of osteogenic loading are based on the loading levels seen in high-impact exercise.

How Bone is Made

Bone is built in a two-step process by cells called "osteoblasts." First, the osteoblasts lay down a matrix of a cartilage-like substance called "osteoid." Next, minerals are deposited onto the osteoid, turning it from a flexible matrix of connective tissue into a hard, solid mineralized structure. Sounds simple enough, right?

But our bodies must be careful in determining precisely how much bone they create. Insufficient bone density leaves us prone to injury, while runaway, unregulated bone growth is seen in some diseases, and can cause serious problems of its own.

That's why our bodies rely on us to "tell" them how much bone density we need, through osteogenic loading.

Wolff's Law & Impact Emulation

In gymnastics and other high-impact sports, we experience osteogenic loading of many times our normal body weight only for an instant. The speed of the increase and decrease of this force is part of what makes it so dangerous: most adult bodies simply are not built to handle such rapid deceleration without tearing or snapping.

Artificially emulating these forces holds the promise, not just of mitigating these dangerous forces, but also of extending the period spent under multiple body weights of osteogenic load indefinitely.

Instead of having a mere instant of compression, we can slowly apply loading equivalent to multiples of the user's body weight, or several G forces. We then maintain this high-impact emulation condition for several seconds. This is a time duration hundreds of times longer than the moment of impact experienced by professional gymnasts after a jump.

Does extending this period of maximum load actually create *more* bone growth than the more dangerous microsecond loading seen in high-impact sports?

In the early days of my research, there was only one way to find out: build impact emulation machines, and measure their bone density-increasing performance against the performance of high-impact exercise.

My research gave me three important points to use in creating my Impact Emulation machine:

- Time-under-tension in impact is short in high-impact exercise. The multiples of bodyweight that lead to the development of greater bone mass are delivered for only a fraction of a second per jump.

- The time-under-tension used in an OsteoStrong session is five seconds. This could seem brief to some, but it is a far greater amount of time under tension than the bone compression experienced in the moment of impact in gymnastics.

- Intensity of loading is key to developing greater bone mass. The more intense the stimulation from bone deformation, the greater the response by the body. This is true of all adaptive responses, not just bone. The same principle applies to the growth of muscle strength and neural connections.

- With our osteogenic loading devices, we would strive to provide the highest level of load that was safe for the user - far exceeding the forces experienced in normal high-impact sports outside of the world of professional gymnastics.

- Repetitive loading is not necessary. The bone mass response seen in gymnasts is greater than what is seen in runners, even though they have fewer impacts than that of a runner who takes thousands of steps. This is because the body's bone growth response depends on the *magnitude* of the osteogenic load, not the frequency of repetition.

Frequently I am asked to comment on the clinical observations that have been made with osteogenic loading use. Patients will say, "I see people getting 7 to 8% bone density gains in one year, but is that good? Doesn't regular exercise build bone also?" I am going to attempt to add clarity for those who ask this question:

Over 100 years ago Dr. Julius Wolff proved his theory to be one of the few things in modern medicine to bear the title of "LAW." A law is a simple equation stating how one variable affects another, which is always true.

Wolff's Law (also called mechanotransduction) is just that - a simple statement which is always true. This law determined that:

If loading/force on bone is able to distort the length and shape of bone temporarily, density of the bone will become greater.

The problem we have today is that this law has been oversimplified into a recommendation of "weight-bearing exercise builds bone."

Although this is technically true, it misses the larger point of the law. It's true that weight-bearing exercise builds bone, but the *amount* of bone built also depends on the amount of weight borne in the exercise.

This is crucial in a world where conventional exercises - such as running - apply relatively tiny amounts of force to our bones, and at a relatively high cost of time, energy, and wear-and-tear on our bodies.

What Helps, And How Much?

In 2012, researchers at the University of Bristol (United Kingdom) identified young active males and females and tracked them for the purpose of analyzing how people reach "peak bone mass" which is the highest point of bone density a typical person will have in their life.

The test group was told to wear activity monitors that tracked the level of force transmitted through the hip based on their activity. This allowed scientists to reliably measure the forces they experienced in their usual exercise routines.

The researchers who performed this study determined that the optimal level of force/loading required an impact from a jump of a minimum height of 15 inches or 39 centimeters.

The results of this study showed that individuals who were able to experience vertical impact forces greater than 4.2 multiples of their bodyweight had significantly greater density in their hips, even though these loads were infrequent.[1]

Remember the "4.2 multiples of bodyweight" number. The idea that multiples of bodyweight - not just a slight increase experienced when running - is necessary for optimal bone growth is key to understanding the unique benefits of OsteoStrong osteogenic loading machines.

This was one of the first studies ever done which specifically identified a relevant level of loading that triggers large bone density gains and demonstrated that fewer repetitions of higher load was more effective than more repetitions of a smaller load.

This evidence brought a greater understanding of the elevated peak bone density levels of athletes who engage in high impact sports. But would that help adults to rebuild lost bone density later in life?

The same researchers from Bristol followed up their experiments with 20 females over the age of 60. This test group was placed into aerobics classes that would favor higher impact activity based on their voluntary movement. Force trackers showed that none of

---

1 Deere, K., Sayers, A., Rittweger, J., & Tobias, J. H. (2012). Habitual levels of high, but not moderate or low, impact activity are positively related to hip BMD and geometry: results from a population-based study of adolescents. Journal of bone and mineral research, 27(9), 1887-1895.

these women were able to attain the 4.2 multiples of body weight with their activity in these classes.

None of the women, in fact, were able to generate more than 2.1 multiples of body weight at any point during the study. Though people with low bone density may not require the full 4 multiples of body weight to see some improvement, the results of this study showed that adults who were active in traditional exercise routines likely could not reverse osteoporosis, or avoid it if they entered adulthood with low peak bone density.

I designed the first osteogenic loading device because I could not find any way to reverse my mother's osteoporosis without drugs, which didn't seem very effective and included many unfavorable side effects.

The objective of the device was simple: The benefit of impact without the risk of injury.

Using a collection of peer-reviewed clinical trials, I compared osteogenic loading devices to various types of exercise, and to the most powerful osteoporosis drugs currently approved and still in the research phases. I found that bone density gains as a result of using these devices could range from 7% to over 14% per year - gains exceeding even the newest and most powerful osteoporosis drugs.

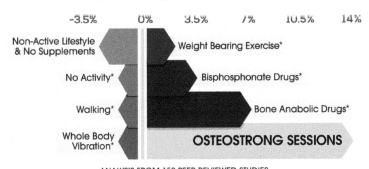

BONE DENSITY ANALYSIS
CHANGES IN BONE DENSITY AFTER 12 MONTHS

| -3.5% | 0% | 3.5% | 7% | 10.5% | 14% |

Non-Active Lifestyle & No Supplements — Weight Bearing Exercise*

No Activity* — Bisphosphonate Drugs*

Walking* — Bone Anabolic Drugs*

Whole Body Vibration* — **OSTEOSTRONG SESSIONS**

ANALYSIS FROM 152 PEER REVIEWED STUDIES
*In each of these studies, participants also took Calcium and Vitamin D3 supplements

Of course, like any procedure or supplement, osteogenic loading is not for everyone. Though it is safe for most people, people with uncontrolled hypertension, muscular dystrophy, no motivation to engage in higher intensity exercise, or the lack of pain-free movement should consider other options.

The machine's activity temporarily increases blood pressure, just like all exercise, and may not be right for people who have medical conditions causing weak muscles or acute pain with exercise.

The good news is, OsteoStrong's side effects are not hidden or time-delayed like those of some medications. Most people can safely try the device and determine if it's right for them. If it isn't, this usually becomes clear immediately and the exercise can be safely stopped.

So if you seek strong bones - either to reverse bone loss, or to build bone mass for athletic performance - consider whether osteogenic loading might be the right biohack for you.

It pairs well with the other biohacks we'll discuss in this book, which take advantage of cutting-edge science to speed up recovery after workouts, improve your body's natural healing abilities, and more.

CHAPTER 2

Superhuman Strength
John Jaquish, PhD & Kyle Zagrodzky

Why Strength Matters

STRENGTH TRAINING ISN'T just for bodybuilders or athletes. Healthy muscles, like healthy bones, are necessary for a healthy life.

Just as a certain level of bone density is needed to avoid serious injury and a host of age-related diseases, so a certain level of muscle strength is needed to avoid serious injury and chronic problems that can be brought on by the conditions we experience every day.

Muscles, after all, aren't just good for lifting weights or performing feats of strength. They lift our bodies out of bed every day, hold our spines in a (hopefully!) healthy position while we sit or stand for hours at work, and play a crucial role in protecting nerves, tendons, ligaments, and cartilage from deterioration.

Insufficient "core strength" - the strength of the muscles in our backs, chests, and bellies which surround our spine and internal organs - can result in dangerous spinal degeneration, pinched nerves, torn tendons and ligaments, cartilage degeneration, trouble standing and walking, and vulnerability to debilitating injury as we get older.

Many of us probably view these as age-related conditions which can't be avoided - but many "symptoms of aging" *can* be avoided with proper exercise and muscular maintenance throughout life. That's why building muscle is just as important for our health as building bone.

This is a rapidly increasing health concern for doctors, as our increasingly sedentary and computer-based lifestyles mean we exercise less in the course of our daily lives. As levels of naturally occurring exercise fall, intentional exercise must be added to our routines to avoid serious health problems as we get older.

Once, children spent most of their childhoods running and playing outside. Sports and physical activities were the most common pastimes. Even for adults, many professions involved physical labor. Jobs often required frequent walking, lifting, stretching, and moving the body in different positions helped to keep our bodies strong and ward off age-related degeneration.

But today, most people of all ages spend most of their time sitting in front of computer screens. From childhood until retirement, we are encouraged to learn, work, and consume entertainment by sitting still without using our muscles at all.

A Crisis of Strength

We mentioned in the last chapter that bone gain and strength gain are deeply interrelated. Your bones and muscles function side-by-side, and depend on each other to function. Because of this, they also respond to similar stimuli which tell them that they must grow to handle more force.

When children play, they often run and jump, and sometimes fall down. This impact stimulus on their bodies is, as described in the jump-training analysis paper, a far larger load than that of their own body weight.[2]

As discussed in our chapter on bone strength, this multiple bodyweight loading increases both their bone mass, and, in a specific way, their muscular mass.

The loads they are receiving are not sustained or repetitive; therefore, they don't resemble the forces encountered in repetitive weight training. Instead, these loads stimulate myofibril development - the development of the power-generating proteins that give us muscle strength - the same way they stimulate bone development. They create a very brief, but very strong force that tells the body that more bone and muscle are needed.

The running, jumping, and the general mechanical impact loading on a child's body eventually evolves into a less active behavior pattern.

With increasing concerns about accidental childhood injury among parents, decreasing recess and gym time allowed by schools, and increasing availability of electronic entertainment, children today have less active lifestyles even in early childhood than those of decades past.

Muscle development can continue in explosive fashion well into adulthood in an athletic individual who is using weights, performing distance running, and doing other athletic activities. But this is not most of the adult population. This means that very few individuals will receive the stimulus for muscle development beyond childhood or young adulthood if they don't participate in high-impact activity.

From the perspective of health, wellness, and athletic performance, muscle development is a variable that needs to be maintained. However, until now there has been no practical way

---

2 Marcus, R. (1996). Skeletal "impact" of exercise. The Lancet, 348(9038), 1326-1327.

to provide multiple body weights of force and stimulate this adaptive response without adopting an intense weight-training routine, which may not be safe for all adults.

An individual who can create a great amount of muscle development can place larger amounts of mechanical loading on the body. But in traditional modalities, this is usually done by increasing force on the body in a rapid and uncontrolled fashion, which can be dangerous for older people.

Because they're triggered by similar stimuli - strong forces that tell our bodies we need to be able to handle heavier loads - bone density and muscular performance can be directly related. The same osteogenic loading forces that stimulate new bone growth can also stimulate new muscle growth.

Let's see exactly how that works.

The Physiology of Strength

Just like with building bone, the basic mechanism behind building muscle is very simple. We use our muscles to the point of exhaustion as a way of "telling" our body that we need more of them.

By lifting the heaviest possible weights or taking gymnastics classes, we tell our muscles that the strength we have right now isn't enough, and we need more of it. Our body then releases chemical messengers which "tell" our muscles to make the proteins they need to become stronger.

If we're really serious about muscle growth, we make sure to eat lots of protein in our diets, so that our muscles will have plenty of raw materials to construct the maximum possible number of new components for our muscles while these growth signals are being released.

The principle is simple. But at a biochemical level, this process is extremely complex. These complexities cause many of the frustrations experienced by exercisers today.

Muscle cells are intricate machines, made up of many molecular "parts" which perform different tasks such as turning fuel into energy and exerting raw mechanical force.

It turns out that the ways we train our muscles can influence which of these parts are strengthened or multiplied. This in turn determines what the muscles we end up with look like, and what they can do.

As you learn more about growing muscle and getting fit, you'll find many training routines that seem contradictory. That's usually because these trainers are trying to accomplish different goals. Someone who wants to increase strength rapidly won't have much use for a bodybuilder's routine, nor will a bodybuilder have much use for a competitive weightlifter's guide.

Why is that? Bigger muscles are stronger muscles, right? Well, not necessarily.

In this chapter, we'll use biology to give you a groundwork for how to achieve two major goals: muscle strength, and muscle size. We'll also explore how osteogenic loading devices can allow you to "hack" strength growth by providing high-intensity exercise to all of the major muscle groups in the body quickly, easily, and safely.

This will allow you to decide how to distribute your training time and energy between the hidden core strength muscles that are necessary for feats of strength and injury risk reduction, and visually prominent muscles that give a great cosmetic effect.

No matter what kind of training you are using, lifting weights and eating more protein should result in gaining some muscle mass. In general, exercising is always better than not exercising.

But over time, you may start to notice that you aren't seeing change as quickly as you'd like. You may realize that your colleagues-in-iron are getting results faster than you, or that you've "plateaued" and are no longer seeing gains in strength or size.

You might find that your bulging muscles don't have the strength to carry out high athletic performance, or that despite gaining immense strength, you don't have the defined physique you're looking for.

That's the time to read up on training and learn the science of muscle building.

One guide might tell you that just like with bone growth, the best way to build new muscle is to lift heavier weights for fewer repetitions. This is what tells your body that your current muscle strength just isn't enough to cope with the loads you have to lift, and that your muscles need to become stronger.

This guide might tell you that you need to focus on compound lifts that exercise many muscle groups so that your strength gains are "functional" and your ability to perform feats of strength isn't held back by a weak muscle group somewhere in your body.

But then there's another guide that says something quite different. This guide tells you to isolate your muscles during training and focus on just one muscle group to cause the maximum muscle exhaustion and, subsequently, maximum growth.

And while you're at it, you need to focus on higher repetition ranges rather than higher weights because really, the only thing that matters is "time under tension." This guide might explain that more time under stress means more muscle growth, while increasing the amount of weight you lift may not make your muscles bigger.

So, who's right? Or are they both right - but for different goals and purposes?

What's Your Fitness Destination?

To know the best way to reach any destination, you must first know where you're going.

When people start athletic training, they usually have some sort of goal in mind. "I want to look a certain way," or "I want to be able to do a certain thing."

What's your fitness destination?

Do you want to reduce your risk of premature death or dementia as you get older? Do you want to have the physique of a bodybuilder or a model? Do you want to be able to perform amazing feats of strength and endurance?

All of those are within your grasp - but there's a different path to achieving each one. How you divide the time and energy you spend exercising will determine your results.

This might sound obvious, but it's something that a lot of people don't consider before they start working out. They just say they want to be "fitter," and grab the first advice guide they see promising any kind of fitness gains.

But what is "fitter" to you? What kinds of changes do you want to see in your body? How do you want to look? What do you want to be able to do? Your answer may be very different from that of a marathon runner, a bodybuilder, or a professional model.

Do you want to feel healthier and have more energy? Do you want to have huge, rippling muscles? Do you want to be able to lift heavy loads, or accomplish feats of gymnastic excellence?

Why do you train?

Is it because you want to be a kind of superhero? In that case, you'll be well suited to a GPP system like CrossFit. This stands for "General Physical Preparedness" and basically means that you're strong and fit across the board and therefore able to defend yourself during a zombie apocalypse.

Maybe you want to look jacked or be able to lift heavy weights. Maybe you want to be leaner, stronger, and more flexible. In this case whole-body exercises like vinyasa yoga might give you the lean strength without bulky size gain that you're looking for.

Or maybe you just want to be a little fitter and healthier so you can be a good influence for your children and be a more active and engaged parent.

In each of these scenarios, the type of training you're going to do is going to be completely different. There will be different tools and exercises that can help you gain cardiovascular health and endurance, flexibility and range of motion, core strength for postural support and injury prevention, bulky muscles for cosmetic purposes, super-strength for lifting weights, and more.

But whatever your desired fitness goals, osteogenic loading can help optimize your gains and prevent injury by ensuring that your bones and muscles are operating at maximum capacity. They do this by loading them with multiples of your body weight.

In this book we'll explain how to accelerate any fitness goal that might be on your map with osteogenic loading. We'll start by discussing a primary goal for good health and athletic prowess alike: gaining muscle strength.

Strength Gain, And How It Works

Most of us could benefit from gaining strength. Whether we're preparing to compete in the Olympics or preparing to cope with the health risks of sitting for long hours in an office chair, increasing our muscles' ability to exert force means increasing our ability to handle the tasks life throws at us.

Ideal health demands that our muscles be able to quickly and easily exert the force necessary to catch ourselves in a fall, or protect our spines during a long work day or a challenging commute. Ideal athletic performance requires the very same.

I want to take a moment here, for purposes of medical clarity, to specify what we mean when we say "muscle" in this chapter. Like most health and fitness resources, when we say "muscle," we'll be referring specifically to the skeletal muscle that produces voluntary movement of your body by pulling on your bones and moving them around. This includes all visible muscles such as biceps, triceps, abs, etc..

Skeletal muscle is not the only type of muscle you have. In fact, different types of muscle cells are found throughout your body in multiple organs, including the heart, arteries, and digestive system, and some of these are also strengthened by exercise. But we can't see these or lift weights with them, so for purposes of this book, we'll be referring to "skeletal muscle" when we say "muscle."

Muscle works by turning the energy you get from food and oxygen into physical movement. Our body produces fuel for our muscles and *all* of our cells in organelles within each and every one of our cells called mitochondria. These mitochondria combine the air we breathe with the food we eat and with the light that hits our skin to produce a fuel molecule called ATP.

We'll talk more about our mitochondria later, in our section on red light therapy. For now, what's important to remember is this fuel called ATP. It's what fuels the actual mechanism of your muscle strength: the contracting of your myosin strands. Think of ATP as the "gasoline" your body needs to operate the biological winches that are your muscles.

In this analogy, myosin is both the chain and engine of your winch. It is a protein which contracts automatically when fueled by ATP, meaning that the quantity and quality of myosin you have determines how much total force your muscles are capable of exerting.

Your quantity and quality of myosin determines how effectively your back muscles support your spine, how effectively you can catch yourself in a fall, how much weight you can deadlift, how powerfully you can launch yourself away from the ground when running or jumping, etc..

Myosin is a long, strong protein used by your muscle cells to pull on your bones. When myosin relaxes, your arm, leg, spine, etc. becomes long and flexible. When it pulls tight, your bicep curls, your knees bend, and all muscle movement arises.

Just like with bone, the amount of myosin our body produces and maintains depends on how much muscle strength our body thinks we need. And just like with bone, the only way to "tell" our body to make more myosin, or more muscle strength, is to use our muscle strength regularly.

Some of you might now be thinking: "Wait. If our body decides how much myosin to make based on how much demand we place on our muscles, doesn't that mean that osteogenic loading devices can *also* be used to build myosin and muscle strength?"

If you're thinking this, congratulations! You're right!

As mentioned in the previous chapter, strength of muscle *and* bone is necessary to withstand and exert force in osteogenic loading. Osteogenic loading is most *uniquely* beneficial for bone growth, since it's harder to deform hard bone tissues and trigger their growth in everyday weight lifting exercises.

But osteogenic loading *also* accomplishes the same effect as a set of high-weight, low-repetition weight lifting. Which is exactly the kind of weight lifting recommended to build muscle strength.

This makes osteogenic just as much of a biohack for functional muscle strength gains as it is for the functional bone strength that prevents injury. In creating a machine to exert maximal force on the body using minimal time and effort, I'd inadvertently created a machine which *also* augmented the kind of strength needed for feats of athletic prowess in addition to merely avoiding injury in osteoporosis.

Because real strength is "functional" - it doesn't depend just on the strength of *one* component in your body, but rather on the strength of *several* components all working together to exert force and accomplish movement - we're going to take a few moments here to discuss each of the several important anatomical features which all need to be strengthened for functional strength gain to occur.

Functional Strength Gain: Bones

As discussed in the previous chapter, "Unbreakable Bones," weak bones are more than a risk factor for debilitating injury. They're also a limiting factor in athletic performance.

When our bones are weak and soft, they're easily deformed and fractured. This condition can be surprisingly common in a society where sedentary lifestyles are the norm, and many people's dietary choices in childhood and beyond are less than the peak of nutritional excellence.

And when our bones are easy to break, our bodies simply won't allow us to build up very much strength or engage in much athletic activity. After all, it would be dangerous for us to exert more force than our bones could handle while lifting weights, running, jumping, or doing any other sort of activity. The process of neural inhibition ensures that our muscles never become functionally stronger than our bones.

It's for this reason that I recommend that every single person who is considering enhancing their strength, whether for reasons of health or athletic performance, adds the use of osteogenic loading devices to their training routine.

Routine osteogenic loading using a properly certified device is incredibly quick and easy, and it guarantees that your strength won't be unnecessarily limited by weak bones as a result of advanced age or poor bone development in childhood.

There's no good reason - not even comfort or convenience - *not* to use this powerful technology to ensure that your bone growth is optimized, removing a potential limiting factor in your muscle growth.

Functional Strength Gain: Myosin

Muscles and bones work together to produce functional strength. That's why bone strength is so important to our ability to create and exert force. It's also why muscle strength and bone strength can both benefit from the same osteogenic loading exercises.

If you're a competitive weight lifter, you know the fastest road to gaining functional muscle strength. To "tell" your body it needs to make more myosin, you have to overload the myosin you already have by lifting extremely heavy loads - say, multiples of your body weight - on a regular basis.

When you lift more weight than your myosin can easily handle on a regular basis, your body releases a signal to tell your muscles that you need more myosin. Just like with bone growth, your body then produces more myosin - thicker chains and a higher-horsepower engine for your muscles - in order to meet your need for more strength.

And just like with bone, it's the *size* of the loads you lift, not the number of repetitions or the amount of "time under tension" that yields functional strength gains.

High reps at a low weight *won't* increase the heaviest load you can lift, or your overall strength, very much if at all. It will only increase your endurance - and your muscle size, making you *look* muscular, regardless of your level of strength.

Muscle Size vs. Muscle Strength: An Important Distinction

Growth in muscle size and growth in muscle strength are two different processes, which are only loosely related.

Myosin - the protein that determines how much force your muscles can create or endure - is a fairly small, thin protein. A single myosin chain is only 15 nanometers in width. That means that doubling or tripling the amount of myosin you have, and doubling or tripling the amount of force your muscles can exert in the process, will result in only small amounts of muscle growth.

This means that specialized training for increased strength has little effect on increased muscle size. By contrast, people who train in order to have bigger muscles often experience surprisingly small strength gains, for all of their impressive size.

This is why Olympic gymnast Simone Biles and the world's weight-lifting champions don't look like bodybuilders, despite likely being stronger than Arnold Schwarzennegger. Bodybuilders train for muscle size - not strength.

It's possible to train for both muscle size and strength. But to reach your goals most effectively it is important to know your fitness destination.

Osteogenic loading will help you maximize your muscle strength, but it will do little for your muscle size. In just the same way, exercise routines followed by bodybuilders will help you increase your muscle size and cosmetic appearance, but may not do much to help you gain strength or avoid injury.

It's important to note here that lifting heavy weights *should always be done under supervision in a controlled environment.*

The principle of exerting extreme forces on your muscles through heavy weight lifting is the same as the principle of exerting extreme force through Olympic-level gymnastic feats. The risks of injury are also the same. If your body is not accustomed to handling high forces, it is easy for your body to tear or break. Needless to say, this will eliminate your ability to exercise and potentially to complete your routine everyday life tasks for months at a time.

That's another reason I recommend osteogenic loading to assist in your strength gain. By applying weight in a slow, controlled manner, you can reduce the risk of injury to all parts of your musculoskeletal system while helping your body become accustomed to handling high loads safely.

Functional Strength Gain: Tendons & Ligaments

There's another component of functional strength that is rarely discussed because it isn't glamorous. Tendon and ligament injuries are not as life-threatening as broken bones, nor are tendon and ligament strength associated with having big, bulging, cosmetically attractive muscles.

For this reason, we only talk about tendons and ligaments when something goes wrong. But you may have noticed that when something *does* go wrong with these crucial components of our functional strength, it's devastating news.

Tendon and ligament injuries are among the most feared types of injuries in competitive sports, due to their relatively slow natural recovery rate after injury and the complete inability of our muscles to function without them.

What are tendons and ligaments? Simply put, they're especially strong pieces of connective tissue that connect our muscles to our bones. If our muscles are the winches, our tendons and ligaments are like the hooks that make sure our bones - the load we are pulling when we move - stay connected to our winch, our muscle cells.

If this hook breaks, it doesn't matter how powerful our winch is: it can't actually grasp or move the load we're trying to move. Our muscle strength is now useless.

Tendon and ligament injuries are a huge risk for athletes and people struggling with clinical bone and muscle weakness alike. When they occur they are painful and debilitating, and unlike most muscle injuries they may require surgery to repair.

The good news is, osteogenic loading systems focus on *functional* strength gains. That means they exercise and strengthen your tendons and ligaments at the same time they're working your bones and muscles.

Avoiding risk of tendon and ligament injury is another vital reason to add osteogenic loading to your workout routine, especially if you are just beginning to exercise and build strength after leading a relatively unathletic lifestyle.

Functional Strength Gain: The Neuromuscular Junction

We've talked extensively so far about the machinery that goes into creating functional strength by using muscles to move and stabilize your bones. But there's one thing we haven't discussed: how do our muscles "know" when to contract, and when to relax?

The answer might seem obvious: we tell our muscles what to do. Our brains control the actions of our hands, feet, arms, and legs. They tell our muscles how to move, when to tense, and when to relax and release.

But at a biochemical level, how does that actually work?

You may have learned in school that our spinal cords and nerves connect our muscles to our brains. Nerve signals originate with thoughts, feelings, and intentions in our brains. From our brains, these biochemical signals called "action potentials" are carried through our spine and our peripheral nerves to tell our muscles what to do.

This is one major reason why protecting our spine from injury by ensuring good bone and muscle strength is so important. When our spines are compressed or injured, as can happen from such mundane tasks as "sitting in front of the computer too much," the nerves that transmit signals from our brains throughout our body can be impaired too.

Severe spinal degeneration, which can arise either from an overly sedentary or an overly strenuous lifestyle, can be mobility-threatening. Spinal bone and muscle degeneration can require braces or surgeries to fix, which may still fail to restore function to damaged nerves, which have less capacity to recover from injury than other types of tissue. This is why having adequate strength, especially in our core bones and muscles, is so important.

But that's enough of doom and gloom for the moment. Let's focus on the bright spots. How can you *improve* your nerves' function, and protect them?

As you may have guessed, cultivating core strength and good bone density is key to protecting your nerves and your mobility in the long term. What you may *not* have realized is that, even beyond protecting your nerves, you can also help them grow.

One often-neglected part of our anatomy is called the neuromuscular junction. This is exactly what it sounds like: the point where our nerves meet and communicate with our muscle cells. The neuromuscular junction is the receiving station where the signals from our brains are turned into muscle contraction.

And just like any neural pathway or muscle, the neuromuscular junction is made stronger and more robust through exercise.

Our body's ability to adapt to the demands of our environment is truly remarkable. Our brain cells and peripheral nerves, just like our muscles, actually grow bigger and stronger when they are used.

Increased activity at the neuromuscular junction will actually cause nerve-muscle connections to become stronger over time, and may even lead to the development of more refined and complex neural capabilities by forming new connections altogether.

This is why Dr. Raj Singh was so interested in my work. In just the same way that my osteogenic loading devices exercised bones, tendons, ligaments, and muscles, they also exercised the neuromuscular junction.

By using osteogenic loading machines, Dr. Singh realized that patients could actually increase the strength of their neuromuscular connections. This would translate to more powerful and reliable muscle activation over time, as the brain got more practice communicating with the muscles of the body.

Dr. Singh believed that this could help patients to avoid injury by improving their neuromuscular activation.

This increase in muscle fiber activation by nerves would result in an overall increase in the amount of force the body could absorb and exert, whether when stabilizing the body during a fall or a long work day, or while performing a feat of athletic prowess.

For Muscle Size Growth

All of us want greater strength so that we can reduce our risk of injury, and increase our ability to exert force in times of need or athletic competition. But some of us also want to *look* like superheroes - which turns out to require a different type of training altogether.

I won't go into great detail about how to achieve bulging muscles here, since this is one area of gain that has yet to be truly hacked.

A "jacked" appearance depends on the size of your muscles' "gas tank." The part of the muscle cell called "sarcoplasm" contains energy-generating mitochondria, as well as ions and sugars to help your mitochondria supply your myosin with a steady stream of ATP.

This cellular "gas tank" doesn't affect how strong your muscles are - instead, it determines how much *endurance* they have, or how *long* they can continue to contract. This "gas tank" also takes up more space than your myosin bundles, so it is the key to big, bulging muscles.

That's why "time under tension" is the bodybuilder's mantra. The more repetitions you push your body to complete, the bigger the "gas tank" your muscles will require. These low-weight, high-repetition routines may not increase the total amount of force you can exert at one time, but they *will* increase your muscle's size and stamina.

Many wonderful bodybuilding books exist to tell you exactly how to use this principle to your advantage.

For best results in strength, safety, *and* cosmetic appearance, try combining "time under tension" bodybuilding exercises with osteogenic loading as a hack for strength. If you want to gain strength *without* getting bulky, on the other hand, focus on high-weight, low-repetition exercises like those offered by osteogenic loading.

Fighting Disease: Strength Gain, Diabetes, and Metabolism

One additional benefit of strength gain deserves special mention, because of its great importance for public and personal health. One little-known effect of increased muscle strength is improved metabolism.

In layspeak, that means lower blood sugar, better blood sugar control, and decreased risk of organ damage from high blood sugar.

High blood sugar is an epidemic which is devastating the world today. One in three people are at risk for diabetes in the near future, or already *have* diabetes due to poor blood sugar regulation.

Like cardiovascular disease and other leading killers in the modern world, this is due to a lethal combination of two things: high-calorie, high-carb diets which raise blood sugar; and sedentary lifestyles without muscular action to use that sugar, allowing it to build up in the blood.

Just about everyone has heard from their doctor or from health PSAs that the way to fight high blood sugar is to exercise more and eat fewer carbohydrates (which are made of sugars). However, what you might not have heard is that there's a way to "hack" this, too.

Eating fewer carbs and moving around more is a good idea for everyone's health. But you can get more benefit for the effort you put in by using osteogenic loading to hack your muscle development - and your metabolism.

The key lies in the impact of muscle tissue on our blood sugar levels. Muscle tissue eats up more calories than other types of tissue, even when it's sitting around doing nothing. In fact, this is a major reason why our bodies eat up and discard our muscle tissue so quickly when we don't exercise: our bodies want to reduce the amount of calories we consume just to stay alive, in case food becomes scarce.

This means that when we exercise and increase our muscle

strength, we are also increasing the rate at which our body burns calories and blood sugar *even when we're sitting around doing nothing.*

In 2015, I was able to show significant benefits to diabetic patients as a result of using osteogenic loading technology. By using these machines to strengthen their bones and muscles, patients were increasing the amount of calories their bodies burned each day.

As with all true biohacks, what was remarkable about this was the cost-benefit trade-off. Significant decreases in A1c levels were accomplished in just a few minutes of osteogenic loading per week, with only a tiny amount of effort or exertion.

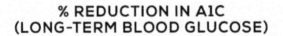

% REDUCTION IN A1C
(LONG-TERM BLOOD GLUCOSE)

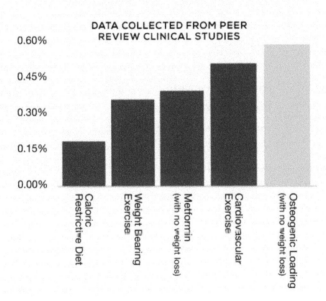

DATA COLLECTED FROM PEER
REVIEW CLINICAL STUDIES

0.60%
0.45%
0.30%
0.15%
0.00%

Caloric Restrictive Diet
Weight Bearing Exercise
Metformin (with no weight loss)
Cardiovascular Exercise
Osteogenic Loading (with no weight loss)

Now, that's not to say you should stop or reduce your existing exercise routine, or eat more carbohydrates, because you started using osteogenic loading devices. To combat the rising global epidemics of weakness, injury, and illness as a result of sedentary lifestyles and poor diet, we must each do all we can to keep our bodies healthy and strong.

But in combination with an active lifestyle and a healthy diet, these machines add *significant* improvements to your metabolic health with almost no added cost in terms of time, effort, and energy.

Where Do I Find Osteogenic Loading Devices?

Osteogenic loading devices are available in some clinics and doctor's offices. However, they may be difficult to locate, and may require prescriptions for use.

We have set out to make these devices more accessible through OsteoStrong - a franchise business which makes osteogenic loading devices affordable to thousands of people seeking to strengthen their bones and muscles.

At present OsteoStrong is growing rapidly, with locations around the world. For this reason we won't attempt to list all locations in this book - chances are that by the time you read it, more locations will have opened around the world.

You can learn more about the OsteoStrong experience and find your nearest Osteostrong location by visiting www.OsteoStrong.me.

CHAPTER 3

Resolve Joint & Back Pain
Kyle Zagrodzky

IN ADDITION TO increased risk of injury and illness, our modern sedentary lifestyles come with another cost that's very important to me personally. That cost is the risk of chronic and severe joint and back pain.

In the modern era, most of us have some form of joint or back pain. Our unbalanced lifestyles - which often feature little to no movement whatsoever, or repetitive, straining movements instead of whole-body exercise - have created an environment where chronic pain is common.

It might seem to you that this kind of pain would be an obstacle to engaging in osteogenic loading. After all, it makes sense that if our joints and muscles are sore, we shouldn't put weight on them. But it turns out that this isn't always true. In fact, osteogenic loading can be a godsend for sufferers of joint and back pain.

I know this firsthand, because I am one of these people.

Some of you may have wondered about this while reading the previous chapters. "How can I use devices that load multiples of bodyweight onto my bones if I already have pain just from the normal activities of daily life?"

The answer lies in a paradoxical discovery: that despite everyday logic seeming to suggest that more load on our joints = more pain, the opposite has proven to be true. For most types of joint and back pain, more loading = less pain. As long as it's done in a safe, controlled, low-impact environment.

The jarring, wear-and-tear effect caused by rapid acceleration and deceleration is the cause of increased joint and back pain in most forms of high-impact, high-loading exercise. But as we've discussed in previous chapters, the osteogenic loading devices invented by John Jaquish, PhD specifically *eliminate* the risk of wear and tear for the safety of osteoporosis and osteoarthritis sufferers.

It turns out that the effects of high loading without high-impact events are miraculous for many sufferers of chronic pain.

Let's explore why the benefits of osteogenic loading for chronic pain are so important to me, personally - and how these benefits work at the biological level.

My Chronic Pain Story

I'm a huge fan of health and fitness. You might have already deduced that, since you know that I've owned heath and fitness franchises in the past and have dedicated much of my life to staying healthy and active.

But at one time in my life, my own ability to be healthy and fit was severely restricted by chronic pain.

Decades of intense high-impact athletics had taken a toll on my bones and joints, and the types of movement I had once loved now resulted in tremendous joint and back pain flare-ups.

Having suffered for decades from chronic joint and back pain from my own sports-related injuries, I have tried many different treatments for relief. Chiropractic care, massages, yoga, ibuprofen - you name it. Each of these *did* relieve the pain - but all were temporary. If I got too busy to return for regular treatments, I'd end up right back where I started.

By my thirties, I had knee pain and could no longer go for a run, pain in my right hip which made walking even short distances difficult, back and neck pain which caused frequent migraine head-aches and kyphosis (hunching of my back), pain in my right shoulder which made lifting more than ten pounds difficult, and pain in my right elbow, which made throwing a ball with my son difficult.

Because a big part of human nature is to avoid pain, the result was that I became less active and less healthy. I began to abbreviate or completely avoid activities that I enjoyed or used to sustain and improve my health.

Living an inactive lifestyle - and feeling that I had no choice about it, because of my pain - made me feel trapped. Was this what the rest of my life was going to be? Slowly becoming less and less active, less and less *able* to be active, for the rest of my days?

I was in a bad place, and my situation was getting worse. I was getting weaker, and slowly gaining excess body fat. I imagined a downward sloping graph in my mind showing a steady decline ahead, and estimated that more serious health issues in my fifties and sixties would be my fate.

Chronic pain is a long-term erosion of both the human spirit and physical health. The physical and mental effects of pain on our nervous systems lead to a gradually degrading quality of life, and premature death due to inactivity and stress.

Years ago, I was on that road. That's why it's so important to me to share this chapter.

I, and thousands of others, have eliminated or greatly reduced our joint and back pain issues with OsteoStrong. If you find yourself in a similar place or know someone who suffers from these challenges, take heart! We have a solution that delivers perpetual relief for many users.

Joint pain of almost any kind comes from the impingement of a nerve between the two joints. After all, only nerves can feel pain - and some of them are placed between our joints intentionally, so that our bodies can tell us when degradation of cartilage or bone makes it dangerous for us to move those joints or place strain on them.

When a joint is in pain, we instinctively protect it by either limiting movement or holding ourselves in a position that reduces the pain. The surrounding muscles work to support the joint or the unnatural, compromised position, often creating muscle soreness or spasms that increase the pain.

Massages are a great temporary relief for this kind of pain, and I personally went for massages almost every week before I tried the new approach we'll discuss here.

Many people also visit chiropractors for relief of back and joint pain. For many years, I was afraid to go to a chiropractor because I thought that there was a chance they could make the pain worse. I was wrong. Chiropractic care was a life-saver for me, and weekly visits would often free me from the pain caused by pinched nerves.

Ibuprofen was a life-saver as well. I never liked taking pills of any kind, and fortunately I avoided more powerful and potentially addictive painkillers. But eventually, I had to admit that I needed something. Ibuprofen was one pill that I was willing to compromise on because it worked when nothing else did.

If I felt my back start to tighten-up, I knew it would lead to a migraine that could last for days. Taking four or five ibuprofen as soon as I felt the beginning of the pain could stop it from spiraling into the dreaded migraine.

I wouldn't leave home without it. I had extra bottles in my car, computer bag, overnight bag and suitcase. I would dread getting on an airplane if I couldn't get an aisle seat, two empty seats, or business class seating. I needed to be able to stand and stretch or walk around if the tightening started up.

Maybe some of this sounds familiar to you. If you are suffering from chronic pain, you seek relief in all of the natural ways - including seeking the ability to engage in natural, healthy movement to help balance unbalanced muscle tension and strain.

But today, my lifestyle is completely different. I can go for a run, engage in resistance strength training, sit in the window seat on an airplane for hours, and enjoy many other activities I once thought were lost to me. I rarely go for massages anymore, and only occasionally go to the chiropractor.

I experience a level of freedom today that I thought I'd never know again, and I've seen many other people report the same. What I am about to share is a biohack - arguably the ultimate biohack - for back and joint pain.

What makes this one so interesting is that it runs contrary to conventional wisdom that these aches and pains arise from overuse, and that the solution is to avoid putting weight on the painful body part.

High-Impact vs. Controlled Loading

In the world of traditional exercise, avoiding loading onto painful joints makes sense. As we've covered earlier, high-impact exercise *can* be dangerous, especially to degraded cartilage and bone which is often the source of the nerve pinching that leads to joint pain.

Low-impact repetitive exercises such as walking can also be bad: these force the painful joints to rub against each other, sometimes becoming even more compressed, without providing any unique stimulation that can lead to joint decompression and regeneration.

So how do we stimulate joint decompression and regeneration? Paradoxically, with more force. But we apply that force in a gentle, controlled manner.

If we think about a joint pinching or impinging a nerve, it stands to reason that decompressing the joint would be the quickest way to relieve the pain. Staying off our joints or stretching them through exercises such as yoga *does* result in pain relief - but it is, more often than not, a temporary solution.

These exercises usually don't stimulate new growth of the bone and surrounding supporting tissue. This means that hours, days or weeks after the exercise is completed, the joint returns to its compromising, nerve-impinging position.

It turns out that a far more effective, more permanent solution for many is to subject the joint to high, self-loaded compression while remaining in a static position.

In other words, you hyper-compress the joint - but don't move it while it is under load. Movement of a joint under high levels of load can lead to painful and damaging grinding of bone on bone or further impingement of the affected nerve.

This sounds contrary to what you might think, right? If compression is the source of joint pain, you'd likely conclude that hyper-compressing the joint could only make things worse.

For most of my life, I agreed with this reasoning. But a published clinical study convinced me to try this approach for myself - and my experience, along with those of thousands of other people I've met, support this finding.

So how do you hyper-compress a joint, loading it with multiples of bodyweight - but without moving it or subjecting it to shock as you would in high-impact exercise?

You may have already guessed the answer. Osteogenic loading devices like those offered by OsteoStrong turn out to deliver this benefit, as well as increased bone density, muscle strength and coordination.

As it turns out, there are three things that happen as a result of an osteogenic loading session, where multiples of bodyweight are placed on the bones and joints.

When a joint is experiencing a loading of force in a static position - that is, not moving - the adaptive response of the central nervous system is to increase blood flow to the joint capsule. A signal is received that the joint is in distress - though it's not actually experiencing any damage, due to its static position - and healing, cushioning blood is sent to fill the joint capsule.

This increase in blood flow will actually cushion the joint, and cause the joint to separate or decompress. This natural decompression frees the impinged nerve, resulting in a reduction or disappearance of the pain almost immediately in many cases.

Often, new clients will notice pain relief that can last for days after their first session, though it may take as many as twelve sessions for the body to sufficiently increase blood flow to the joint capsule to offer even more, long-lasting relief.

The second effect of osteogenic loading devices occurs in the tissue surrounding the joint, such as ligaments, tendons and muscles. In response to extreme loading, as we've discussed in previous sections, both bone and muscle become stronger and able to withstand and generate more force.

Loading makes the supporting tissues stronger. But osteogenic loading often produces different, faster results by safely loading many multiples body weight onto the joint. Without osteogenic loading devices, this is almost impossible to achieve without causing a rapid, uncontrolled impact on the joint.

With repeated loading, the tissue surrounding joints (including muscles, ligaments, and tendons) will become stronger and thick enough to hold the joint in a more consistently decompressed or slightly separated position. This increased ability of surrounding soft tissues to hold the joint in a safe position often frees the pinched nerve, with benefits lasting as long as that strength is maintained.

As a final and unique benefit, the bone in the joint can actually reform and be strengthened if the osteogenic loading is sufficient.

As we discussed previously, clinical research discovered that

4.2 multiples of body weight loading is the minimum dose of pressure needed to trigger an adaptive response from the central nervous system to build bone. This can only be safely achieved in people with existing bone and joint problems through the use of osteogenic loading devices.

Together, increasing blood flow and increasing the density and strength in these tissues (muscle, ligament and tendons, and bone) can greatly reduce or eliminate joint pain in most people.

The exciting news is that this benefit is available to most people who may have difficulty with traditional exercise, like I once did.

One important caveat is that osteogenic loading has *not* been shown to generate new cartilage in joints. The loading can increase blood flow to existing cartilage and strengthen surrounding supportive tissues, but it will *not* repair torn or damaged cartilage. This means that people with torn or damaged cartilage may experience reduced pain and reduced risk of future injury as a result of the other benefits of osteogenic loading, but will not experience cartilage repair.

Similarly, osteogenic loading can relieve pain in cases of arthritis, and may even help to rebuild bone in cases of osteoarthritis. But osteogenic loading will not *cure* the underlying diseases in cases of rheumatoid arthritis, which is caused by a viral infection or autoimmune response.

Because the origin of rheumatoid arthritis is not in the bone or muscle itself, strengthening bone will not necessarily cause the symptoms to vanish or halt the disease process. But it can help to fight the symptoms by decompressing and strengthening the joint through the mechanisms discussed above.

OsteoStrong's osteogenic loading devices have been shown to be very helpful for people with replaced hips and knees, as well. Sessions can strengthen the internal bone structure, called trabecular bone. This is the part of the bone that grips the prosthetic joint, helping it to function better and reducing the risk of injury.

Osteogenic loading has even been recommended by doctors prior to joint replacement surgery, to help strengthen the bone by stimulating new growth in the trabecular bone to which the implant will be attached. Having stronger trabecular bone helps the surgeon by creating a better foundation to attach the implant, and reduces the risk of later injury.

The good news is, using OsteoStrong devices is easy to do and only takes a few minutes of sweat-free effort once a week.

The latest and most powerful version of the OsteoStrong system includes four proprietary devices which allow users to engage in brief and simple loading of their joints in optimal positions in order to experience high levels of force, often many multiples of their own body-weight.

Loading *more* weight onto aching joints may sound crazy to anyone, let alone someone living with joint and back pain. But this approach has been shown to be incredibly effective, with between one to twelve sessions offering relief to many people who have lived with chronic pain for decades.

Keeping up with regular weekly sessions after the cessation of pain will continue to strengthen the bone, muscle, and surrounding tissues. This provides more structure and support to the joint, helping to prevent future injury. As discussed in the bone density section, these exercises actually have the power to reverse what was historically assumed to be the unavoidable effects of aging.

If you're like me and you experience decades of pain all but disappearing after a few short sessions, it feels like a miracle.

Later in this book, we'll discuss additional health measures which have been shown to improve healing of problems related to bone density, inflammation, injury, and more.

So read on to learn biohacks for your metabolism and overall health - and to learn about the specific benefits of these biohacks for bone strength, injury healing, and overall health and well-being.

CHAPTER 4

Biohack Your Body With Pulsed Electromagnetic Fields
Greg Musser, ND

A Note From Kyle Zagrodzky

I AM A huge fan of this particular biohack. It's easy to implement and has a wide range of health benefits.

There aren't many biohacks that simply allow you to sit-and-get without expending effort or changing your behavior, but this is one of them. This chapter is going to jump into a lot of the science and benefits of Pulsed Electromagnetic Fields (PEMF).

The basic premise is that our bodies have a certain electromagnetic frequency that's similar to the earth's frequency. By spending time inside, wearing rubber-soled shoes and surrounded by the electro-smog of mobile phones and wifi signals, our body's frequency becomes misaligned. This has consequences for our health and cellular function.

Spending time every day on bare ground, with bare feet can help realign our frequency to the earth. There are many documented health benefits of doing this every day. PEMF seeks to emulate the earth's electromagnetic field but with more power, allowing us to reap the benefits of this frequency with more intensity and less time investment than traditional earthing or grounding.

PEMF has been used for decades, ever since electrical technology became widely available. But this technology is only now gaining broader acceptance in the medical community, due to science's ever-increasing understanding of how our bodies work and how they interact with the world around us.

The devices which generate these helpful fields of energy are seemingly simple, but have such an interesting impact on health that explaining how and why they work warrants much more than a single chapter. We will cover some of the most interesting aspects here.

PEMF devices are a biohack that shouldn't be underestimated, so I encourage you to take the time to really understand what's contained in this chapter. We'll go into some technical details here about what electromagnetic fields actually are, how they're created, and how they interact with your body everyday both indoors and outdoors.

This might feel a bit like being back in school in science class at times, but it's all to help you really understand what benefits PEMF holds for you if you add this biohack to your daily routine.

In this chapter, you'll learn how PEMF devices can:

- Reduce inflammation throughout your body

- Increase your rate of healing from injury and illness

- Improve circulation throughout your body

- Improve your bone health and healing

- Improve your overall mood and sense of well-being

The Bioenergetic World

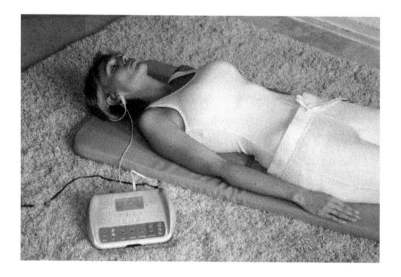

We live each day surrounded by electromagnetic fields. You may think I mean those generated by your computer and other devices - but those aren't the only ones.

Natural electromagnetic fields are generated by the Earth, the Sun, and weather processes. We live in a bioenergetic world, and we always have.

The Earth generates an extremely strong magnetic field thanks to the natural movement of metals in the Earth's crust. Without this magnetic field, we would die: it plays the vital role of deflecting cosmic radiation and protecting life on Earth. It also permeates every cell of our bodies, all the time.

Wind and water currents move past each other just like the metals in the Earth's mantle, producing their own electromagnetic fields and charges. The most dramatic evidence of this is lightning - a huge electrical current that occurs to balance electrical currents between the earth and sky during storms.

By treating this as a merely interesting fact - not a biologically important one - scientists missed a vital part of the world we live in for many decades.

As we'll learn in the pages to come, the cells of our body create electromagnetic currents. Actions we take to support or disrupt these currents can affect our health. We'll also learn that many particles in our bodies are electrically charged, and respond to electromagnetic fields. Under natural circumstances we move through electromagnetic fields which interact with our own every day.

This means that the body not only has a vascular system and a nervous system - but also a less obvious, but very important electromagnetic system.

Electromagnetic Fields In Our Bodies

The human brain consists of about 100 billion nerve cells, called neurons, with trillions of connections between them.

That means there are more neural connections in a cubic centimeter of brain tissue than there are stars in the Milky Way galaxy! This immense neural network is responsible for all of human experience.

Messages about what we are thinking, feeling, and experiencing are transmitted from one neuron to another with the help of electricity. When our millions of neurons communicate simultaneously, their patterns of electrical activity can be measured with an EEG. Today, EEGs can be used to diagnose whether the brain's electrical activity is healthy - or whether it is a source of illness.

Similar electrical activity keeps our bodies healthy every day. This electrical activity that keeps our cells alive naturally creates its own magnetic fields.

Sounds weird, right? But whenever electricity flows, charged particles and molecules like ions are being moved. This means that a proportional magnetic field is created according to Ampere's law which describes the relationship between electric charge and magnetic fields.

This is not magic, but electromagnetic physics. And it's not just an interesting fact: it's one we can use to hack our own moods, health, and healing.

The biomagnetic fields of our bodies are measurable. Magnetoencephalography (MEG) and magnetocardiography (MCG) measure the magnetic fields generated by the electrical activity in the brain and heart, and can also be used to diagnose problems with these organs.

But how exactly does the body create and control these magnetic fields? And, more importantly, what can we do for our bodies if we learn how to influence them?

The Role of the Cell Membrane

The "skin" of our cells is called the cell membrane. Just like the skin of our bodies, this membrane is responsible for keeping our cells' insides where they're supposed to be, and keeping toxins, pathogens, and other dangerous invaders out of our cells.

For decades, scientists have known that it's the job of the cell membrane to carefully "decide" what does or doesn't get to enter a cell. The cell membrane must take in chemicals like water, sugar, fatty acids, amino acids, vitamins, and minerals to fuel the cell's growth. It must keep out substances like toxins, bacteria, and anything the cell already has too much of. Even too much water can be dangerous if allowed to cross the cell membrane.

The cells use this special property of the cell membrane - its selective permeability, or ability to "decide" what gets in and out of a cell - to create electrical voltage.

This voltage is called the "transmembrane potential." It is the difference between the electrical charge of the inside and outside of a cell.

This potential is created by the cell membrane, which uses the energy it gets from food and oxygen to pump ions - atoms, mostly sodium and potassium, which carry a positive electric charge when dissolved in water like they are in our bodies - in and out of the cell.

As these ions are pumped, the inside of the cell becomes positively charged compared to the outside. When our cells "want" to send a signal, they open gates in the cell membrane that allow charged particles to flow in and out rapidly. The resulting voltage changes help cells to work together, and to move necessary ingredients in and out of their cellular bodies. This effect is so strong it can be used to concentrate substances inside cells in seemingly unnatural ways, against their natural diffusion gradients.

It is this effect of electrical voltage and charge difference that keeps our cells alive. It can also be used by our cells to send signals, such as nerve signals, or the signal that new bone growth is needed.

This effect is so important that it explains why our cells begin to die within mere minutes of oxygen deprivation: without oxygen, our cells can't make the ATP necessary to power the proteins that move ions around in order to maintain this electrical charge.

Without this crucial ability to transport and signal, our brain cells begin to die and our heart soon stops beating.

This operation of building up electrical charge is what allows us to think and feel, what keeps our heart beating, and what allows most of the cells in our body to perform their essential functions.

Now that we've seen the extreme importance of electromagnetic fields to the functioning of our cells and bodies, it's easy to understand why electromagnetic fields can have profound health benefits when used to support and reinforce healthy cellular activity.

What is a Pulsed Electromagnetic Field (PEMF)?

With the power of technology, we can create electromagnetic fields artificially simply by running electricity through a copper coil.

These fields exert influence on electrically charged particles, and they can be used to support the healthy movement of charged particles within our cells.

PEMF stands for Pulsed Electromagnetic Field. Usually, the PEMF is calibrated to pulse at roughly the same rate as healthy human cells, or at a resonant frequency that supports them (we'll speak more about resonant frequencies soon).

These magnetic fields are capable of moving charged particles - and of strengthening or weakening the action potentials of cells that are exposed to them.

Magnetic fields affect the behavior of any other charged objects near the field. This is the fundamental basis for their therapeutic use. Since our bodies are electric, external magnetic fields interact with the normal electromagnetic fields produced by the body. A magnetic field passing through our whole body will have an electromagnetic effect on each of our 70-100 trillion cells.

As a result, magnetic fields act in a basic and fundamental way on molecules and tissues. They affect the most basic functions of all cells - human, animal, and plant included.

The weight of clinical research showing benefits of PEMF for a dizzying range of health conditions is enormous. And we are now able to take advantage of these benefits, either by purchasing a PEMF device for our homes or by visiting a facility that offers PEMF sessions on-site like most OsteoStrong centers.

One big benefit to magnetic field therapy is that it can produce big changes inside cells - without being invasive, penetrating, or painful. Because PEMF therapy uses invisible, painless magnetic fields as a means of stimulation, it can induce charges deep in the body. This procedure is non-invasive, safe, and totally without discomfort.

The only affects the user generally notices are the benefits, which can range from improved mood, energy, and peace of mind, to decreased growth of cancer cells or faster healing of an injury.

Sound too good to be true? In the pages to come, we'll be citing the peer-reviewed clinical research that discovered these remarkable results. We'll even include a link to more assembled research online, because there was just too much to present it all here.

One reason PEMFs are so gentle is that they work by inducing ionic shifts within your tissues. This means they can only produce as much charge and current as the tissues are naturally capable of.

You're not "zapping" your cells with electricity, so tissues cannot be overcharged by PEMF. They can only be supported, aligned, and harmonized by PEMF pulses within the biological window - or in some cases interfered with by disruptive "electrosmog" from other electronic devices.

The increased prevalence of "electrosmog" from household devices, along with our decreasing exposure to the healthy, natural electromagnetic fields of the Earth are two reasons why people may need PEMF support for optimal health and healing, even though our ancestors didn't in the past.

This is also one reason why PEMF is sometimes called high-tech "grounding," or "Earthing" - these fields are designed to amplify healthy electromagnetic activity and simulate the healthy exchange of ions and electromagnetic charges that our bodies naturally get when we spend time in direct physical contact with the Earth.

So what exactly do these healthy, supportive PEMFs do for your health?

Revitalize Your Membrane Potential

PEMFs enhance the function of cell membranes by helping restore healthy transmembrane potential and revitalizing the cell.

This is especially true for the sodium/potassium and calcium ion channels in a cell. These are essential for keeping cells alive and allowing them to function normally. The best-studied effects of PEMFs are the effects they have on the activity of these ion channels.

The positive effects of PEMFs on the calcium channels appear to be responsible for most of the physiological effects of PEMFs, including enhanced healing of injuries and anti-cancer action.

In short, PEMFs promote and support healthy cell membrane activity. This effect is so strong that it has been shown to induce healing in non-healing bone fractures, and to strengthen healthy cells while disrupting the growth of unhealthy cells with unhealthy membrane potentials such as cancers.

We'll discuss more of the specific health benefits PEMF has been shown to support in the pages to come.

The Principle of Resonance

Resonance is a principle discovered by Galileo Galilei in 1602 when he studied the motion of a pendulum. It describes the tendency of a system to oscillate - or move back and forth - with a maximum amplitude at a specific frequency.

The principles of resonance can be applied, not just to the motions of a pendulum, but also to sound waves, electromagnetic waves, and any sort of rhythm such as the rhythm by which our cells change their voltage and electrical charge.

If you apply the correct frequency to a system - called the system's "resonant frequency" - the results will be self-reinforcing and will be much greater than the results from applying any other frequency.

A well-known example from daily life is the children's swing, which behaves just like a pendulum. If you push the swing exactly at the moment of the natural oscillation interval (its resonant frequency), the swinging motion amplifies more and more up to the maximum amplitude. An attempt to amplify the rocking motion outside of the resonant vibration results in a weakening or even halting of the movement.

A more humorous story is that of a Japanese building, which experienced significant shaking and evacuated out of concern that an earthquake was occurring. The shaking happened because a single exercise class on one of the building's floors had aligned with the building's resonant frequency while exercising to a new song.

The greatest possible resonance effect is achieved when something resonates exactly in synchrony with its natural fundamental frequency, and thereby amplifies the self-oscillation.

Resonance and the Human Body

Cells in the human body oscillate naturally. Action potentials and the "swinging" of a cell's electrical charge act very much like the physical swinging of a pendulum.

Just as with a swing or office building, force can be applied in ways that reinforce the rhythm of our cells' healthy electromagnetic activity - or in ways that disrupt it, depending on the frequency of the forces. Electromagnetic pulses tuned to the right frequency can enhance the life-sustaining self-oscillation of the cell, while "electrosmog" may interfere with the cell's natural polarity.

In addition, the cell's receptors for neuropeptides ("chemical messengers" that deliver messages between cells, like those mentioned in other chapters) oscillate as well. Electromagnetic waves generate resonances which can have a positive effect on many functions within the cell, and on the cell's surface where chemical messages are received and sent.

On average, the human body consists of about 70 to 100 trillion cells. Each cell has about 1 million neuropeptide receptors. These receptor proteins send and receive messages to and from other cells, including signals that promote healing, action potentials (including those by which our brain tells our muscles to activate), and other cellular "behaviors."

Applying an electromagnetic signal at the correct frequency stimulates a cell's receptors and leads to an amplification of these signals, and the improvement of numerous cell functions as a result.

Induction of an electromagnetic field throughout the human body stimulates and enhances intercellular communication, positively and sustainably affecting bodily functions. Extremely low frequency and very low frequency electromagnetic pulses, such as those generated by PEMF devices, accomplish this positive effect.

But higher frequencies - such as those generated by cell phones, wireless technologies, and power lines - can interfere with these natural cellular biomagnetic rhythms. Instead of reinforcing and synchronizing a cell's healthy activity, they disrupt and weaken the cell.

The latest generation of intelligent magnetic resonance pacing systems uses extremely low and very gentle frequency and intensity ranges, which are in the resonance spectrum of the human cells.

Today, the IMRS / Omnium1 PEMF systems from Swiss Bionics are the best example of high-precision, computer-controlled generation of well-defined electromagnetic waveforms in order to achieve a maximum cell resonance.

As part of our continued effort to make the very best in health and biohacking available to the public, we have made these machines available for use by members at most OsteoStrong locations.

Putting PEMF in OsteoStrong clinics is an especially good fit because it turns out that one of the health benefits of PEMF is stronger bones, and faster bone healing. We'll explore the powerful clinical evidence supporting this benefit, and its precise mechanism of action, later in this chapter.

The Biological Window

Dr. Ross Adey, an Australian-born professor of anatomy and physiology working at UCLA School of Medicine, coined the term "biological window" to describe the frequency at which electromagnetic fields support the metabolism of cells rather than interfering with them.[3]

Adey measured the calcium output of brain cells in rabbits to demonstrate that this beneficial effect could only be triggered using very low magnetic field intensities and a specific low (16 Hz) frequency. Since Dr. Adey's initial discovery, the energy medicine literature has shown strong scientific consensus that biological windows are important.

A biological window is a range or spectrum of electromagnetic frequencies which are readily accepted by the body and converted into positive physiological responses. This means that there is a range of intensities and frequencies for which the tissue is especially receptive.

Magnetic fields pass through the body without creating any direct sensation. But when magnetic field impulses of the correct frequency permeate the body, they can resonate with the natural oscillation of cells and organ systems.

To understand what exactly is happening, we have to take a look at the nature of electromagnetic waves like those created by a PEMF device.

Waves always have a specific amplitude (strength) and frequency (wavelength). Waves can strengthen each other, weaken each other, or even cancel each other out.

You've probably seen this if you've ever watched ripples spread out in water. As ripples or waves from different directions meet,

---

3 Bawin SM and Adey WR. 1976. Sensitivity of calcium binding in cerebral tissue to weak environmental electric fields oscillating at low frequency. Proc Natl Acad Sci U S A. 1976 Jun; 73(6): 1999–2003.

they can combine to form larger waves, or cancel each other out to create spots of dead water. This also applies to invisible waves, such as sound waves and electromagnetic waves.

In sound waves, a harmony is always generated when two individual tones meet at exactly the same wavelength. The resulting combination creates a pleasant and amazing sound, which we define as a harmonic sound.

In contrast, we experience disharmony whenever we hear sounds that differ in their wavelengths and do not meet in synchrony, but instead interfere with each other. This is called "dissonance."

Continuing with this example, a so-called musical overtone is created - that is, a brand new frequency of sound - when harmonies are added to the fundamental note. Harmonies must be in perfect, mathematical relationship to produce this mutually supportive effect. The resonance between them produces a whole new frequency, or sound.

These overtones are created by the principle of the resonance characteristics of harmonic frequencies, without these notes being played or sung. This phenomenon is called stochastic resonance.

Similar principles can be seen in the action of electromagnetic waves.

Synchronized oscillation of electromagnetic fields leads to resonance. This means there are frequencies which are not produced directly, but rather arise from the sum of electromagnetic oscillations and their resonant properties with the human cell.

The induction of cell resonance - synchronous, biomagnetic oscillations in our body - is responsible for the biological effect of PEMF, which supports and promotes the initiation and acceleration of the body's own healing processes.

The cell receptors - especially those of already dysfunctional cells - are prompted to resonate with the basic biological frequencies and the harmonic overtones that occur at the same time. The metabolism gets going, and a variety of disturbed functions are balanced, harmonized and optimized. The result is a fundamental and sustainable improvement in overall health.

Harmonic oscillations are frequencies that arise due to the multiplication of the corresponding fundamental frequencies (similar to the overtones in music). For example, rectangular pulses with a frequency of 1 Hz also generate harmonics of 3, 5 and 7 Hz simultaneously. First-generation harmonics, which trigger second-generation harmonics, even have the same force as the original oscillation.

In order to generate resonance, the field strength of the magnetic field (flux density) and the applied, pulsating frequencies combined must be in resonance with the frequency of the body's cells, not in interference with them.

In Swiss Bionics PEMF devices, mathematical probability calculations are used to calculate the optimal resonance phenomena and thus the strongest biological effects with magnetic field therapy.

The resonance effect restores disrupted or abnormal cellular and/or cell receptor oscillations that are vital for metabolic processes, circulation, cell regeneration and the immune system, and the result is an enhanced feeling of well-being.

How Does This Benefit My Health?

Some of the basic actions of a cell are to generate energy, to eliminate waste, to repair and regenerate itself, and to perform its functions for the body as a whole. Brain, heart, lung, liver, and kidney cells each have their own unique function. But it's important that *all* of them be healthy and strong, so that they can perform their functions for our bodies as a whole.

Cells stay healthy by moving "good" substances in and "bad" substances out across their cell membranes. A healthy transmembrane potential is needed for a cell to do this effectively.

In fact, transmembrane potential is so important that roughly

25% of your body's fuel - a full quarter of all the air you breathe and the calories you burn - is devoted to producing ATP which is used to maintain transmembrane potential.

That's how important transmembrane potentials are to life. They are arguably the single biggest investment of energy your body makes in order to stay alive.

Needless to say, this means that supporting and promoting healthy transmembrane potential through PEMF is a big step toward overall wellness for all cells.

Through the increased motion of ions and electrolytes, magnetic fields can help cells regenerate their transmembrane potential faster and strengthen their ability to transmit signals and simply stay healthy and alive.

Can PEMF Prevent Disease?

Cellular injury - the state of a cell when it is not healthy and functioning properly - leads to disease conditions. Magnetic fields have been shown to improve circulation, repair processes, and energy restoration, and to increase special stress proteins in the cells.

These proteins are used to prevent cell breakdown and wear and tear, as well as help speed recovery from injury. Magnetic fields balance cells, tissues and bodily functions at very fundamental levels, even before damage and problems become obvious to you.

What About the Electromagnetic Field from My Computer?

There are distinct differences in the atomic, molecular, and biological effects of magnetic fields at different frequency ranges and energy levels. Electromagnetic fields come in a variety of frequencies and wavelengths, from extremely low frequencies (ELFs) and very low frequencies (VLFs), to microwave frequencies, radio, infrared, visible light, ultraviolet frequencies, and more.

Although all of these forces are made up of the same particles, they carry different energy levels which means that they have different helpful, or destructive effects on cells.

The difference between an extremely low frequency field and a very high frequency field like a microwave can be thought of as the difference between massaging your cells with gentle hands and firing bullets at them. Many other frequencies exist between these energy extremes of force.

These energy levels are not a matter of how strong the field is - they're a matter of frequency, which is different from intensity. Being massaged by many hands is not the same as being shot by one bullet, anymore than being shot by just *one* bullet is similar to a massage.

The frequency and energy levels of the particles is what determines their helpful and harmful ability - not the strength of the field.

This is why even MRI machines - which generate fields 60,000 times stronger than those of the planet Earth - are safe for the people who work around them every day, as long as their safety instructions are followed.

Most magnetic field exposure risk is thought to come from man-made electromagnetic environments, like power lines, cell phones, Bluetooth, WiFi, microwaves, and 5G, often referred to as electrosmog. These fields are not designed to be therapeutic, and may be disruptive to healthy cellular functioning.

If and to what extent this man-made electromagnetic environment is harmful to our bodies is still controversial. Some scientists believe there is not enough evidence that our unnatural electromagnetic modern environment causes harm, while others believe it would be foolish to assume it doesn't.

Most PEMF devices produce frequencies in the ELF to VLF range. Our home-based devices have carefully selected frequencies which mimic the natural electromagnetic fields of our own bodies and of the Earth.

How Fast Does PEMF Work?

Minor imbalances in individual cells can be rebalanced easily before they become an obvious problem. Unfortunately, many people wait until they have significant symptoms and health issues before they seek a doctor or use some kind of wellness device.

By this time, some problems may have become too deep-seated to reverse. Others may require long-term treatment to complete a slow but steady healing process, which may be made faster, but not instantaneous by PEMF.

It is important to be clear that PEMFs are not expected to cure a disease process that is already underway on their own. Their role is to stimulate the various functions of the body so that the body can better support and heal itself. For acute illnesses and injuries, best results can be obtained by combining supportive PEMF with other therapies that attack the disease process or injury in a targeted way.

PEMFs will not make a physical illness or injury vanish immediately. Instead, they may speed up healing time and improve ultimate healing results. As a general rule it's always wise to seek care from doctors for illnesses and injuries, while using general health and wellness measures like PEMF to support and improve the results of medical treatments.

The best medicine is, of course, prevention. Anything we can do to support healthy cellular processes is likely to pay off with better health in the long-run.

What Other Benefits Does PEMF Have?

Clinical research has shown PEMF therapy to be beneficial for a dazzling array of injuries and diseases. We'll discuss the specific documented benefits of PEMF in the pages to come.

If you are happy understanding the general principles by which PEMF helps all cell types, feel free to skip this section.

But if you want to see the clinical research findings that show PEMF's specific benefits in more detail, read on!

PEMFs for Improving Blood Flow & Oxygen

One of the most basic effects of magnetic fields on the body is to increase circulation - especially microcirculation.

The term "microcirculation" refers to blood flow in the smallest vessels. These are composed of arterioles, capillaries and postcapillary venules. Also included are the terminal lymphatics.

These capillaries are so-called terminal flow paths - that is, the vessels are dead ends, which makes it more difficult for blood to move and flow efficiently. They are also some of the most important blood vessels in the body.

The capillaries are where the blood circulation performs its most important task: the exchange of substances between blood and tissue. In the capillaries, blood delivers vital oxygen, fuel, nutrients, and immune proteins to cells, and removes harmful waste products.

In other words, if the microcirculation does not work properly, the supply of oxygen and nutrients, and the removal of carbon dioxide and cellular waste products also don't work properly.

Poor microcirculation makes tissues unhealthy and prone to disease and breakdown. It is poor circulation that can cause necrosis and the need for amputation in people with diabetes, whose high blood sugar can make the blood serum thicker and interfere with blood flow.

Poor microcirculation has been implicated in a number of diseases featuring general deterioration of tissues, and how much blood flow a tissue receives determines its speed of healing from disease or injury.

Red blood cells transport oxygen from our lungs to every cell in our body. Our cells need this oxygen to produce ATP.

A cell's ability to perform its functions for our body, and even to stay alive, depends on having a sufficient supply of oxygen. Impaired oxygen transfer to our cells can mean impaired cell function, and even cell death. Luckily, our body has a huge fleet of red blood cells to deliver the oxygen our cells need.

The number of red blood cells we carry and produce is amazing. We produce more than 200 billion red blood cells per day, which is equivalent to two million per second. These cells make up 70% of all cells in our body.

The blood cell's oxygen deliveries occur mainly in tiny, narrow capillaries. Capillaries are so incredibly small that the red blood cells must be able to change their shape to push through. Unfortunately, a phenomenon called the "Rouleaux effect" can make this process difficult or impossible.

A Rouleaux formation consists of a stack of red blood cells that stick together. It resembles a stack or roll of coins that you might get from the bank, and is therefore commonly referred to as "roll forming." Due to the disc-like shape of erythrocytes, they are predisposed to this type of clumping.

Capillaries can each pass only a single red blood cell - stacks just won't fit through. Therefore, it is necessary to prevent Rouleaux formations from occurring in order to ensure healthy blood flow.

Because PEMF therapy supports healthy cell membrane charge, it has a direct impact on this effect. Healthy, charged red blood cells have similar electromagnetic charges - meaning they'll repel each other and will not stick together. Red blood cells that are struggling to maintain their cell membrane charge, on the other hand, are more likely to stick together.

Apart from preventing the "Rouleaux effect," this separation of red blood cells allows for a larger available surface area for oxygen and nutrient uptake and exchange.

Unwanted coagulation of blood in the blood vessels can range from tiny Rouleaux formations that often go unnoticed, to life-threatening blood clots that can block arteries leading to the heart or brain.

PEMF therapy reduces platelet adhesiveness, reduces fibrinogen - a protein that helps blood clots form - and improves red blood cell deformability, making it easier for blood cells to move through capillaries.

PEMF won't substitute for medication therapy in blood clotting disorders, but it can improve blood flow and cellular oxygenation in healthy people and people who are already being treated to prevent clots. More research is needed to determine if PEMF might also reduce symptoms in people with blood clotting disorders, when used in combination with the necessary medications.

Vasodilation is the dilation of the blood vessels. It comes from the term "dilate" for "to relax" or "to get bigger," and the term "vaso" for "vessel."

In the body, Nitric Oxide (NO) is a powerful "vasodilator," or a chemical that causes blood vessels to open up. Abnormal or decreased production of NO can occur in cases of injury, disease, and poor health. This affects blood flow and other vascular functions.

In a healthy cell environment, blood vessels are constantly producing nitric oxide. In the inner lining of the blood vessels, called the endothelium, nitric oxide serves as a messenger to "tell" the smooth muscle in the blood vessel wall to relax, opening the vessels.

The subsequent increase in blood flow leads to a decrease in both blood pressure and heart rate, since the heart does not have to work as hard to push against the blood vessels' resistance.

PEMFs can stimulate increased release of NO, leading to benefits including improved nutrient transport, increased repair molecules and growth factors, increased oxygen, and more efficient elimination of waste products.[4]

---

4 McKay JC, Prato FS, et al. A literature review: the effects of magnetic field exposure on blood flow and blood vessels in the microvasculature. Bioelectromagnetics. 2007 Feb;28(2):81-98.

PEMFs also positively affect the ability of hemoglobin - the iron-based chemical in red blood cells that binds to oxygen, allowing our cells to carry it - to transport and deliver precious air.

One study of PEMF effects on tissue focused on the effect of magnetic fields on the gas transport function of blood during oxygen deprivation. They found that magnetic therapy changed the hemoglobin molecules from a form that was less reactive to oxygen into a form that was more reactive.

In other words, hemoglobin molecules treated with PEMF were more eager to respond to oxygen in the lungs by binding to it, and more likely to successfully release that oxygen for the use of other cells upon entering low-oxygen blood vessels.[5]

Another study was performed on patients with terminal emphysema - a condition which destroys the lung's ability to expand and contract in order to draw oxygen into the body.

These patients received PEMF therapy (30 minutes per day for seven days) in addition to their usual medical care. The addition of magnetic field therapy improved blood oxygen levels by up to 21%, and all patients reported feeling they had better physical endurance. It is possible that these results would have been even more significant if the treatments were performed earlier in the disease and for a longer period of time.[6]

One of the earlier demonstrations of the benefits of PEMFs to improve oxygenation was made in the early 1990s in Germany with a large PEMF plate.

This experiment found that PEMF benefits were enhanced during periods of high muscle activity, alcohol intake, sleep, or after

5 Muehsam D, Lalezari P, et al. Non-thermal radio-frequency and static magnetic fields increase rate of hemoglobin deoxygenation in a cell-free preparation. PLOS One. 2013 Apr 12;8(4):e61752.

6 Jerabek J, Pawluk W. Magnetic therapy in Eastern Europe: a review of 30 years of research. Publ Advanced Magnetic Research of the Delaware Valley, Chicago, 1996.

inhalation of carbon dioxide - a waste product which we normally breathe out in order to prevent it from reaching toxic levels in our blood. Hyperventilation - increasing air flow through the lungs - and large meals would reduce the level of benefit from PEMF.

In other words, PEMF was especially effective at helping people suffering from less-than-ideal conditions, while people who already had plenty of cellular fuel thanks to a healthy lifestyle, benefitted less from PEMF because their bodies were already working properly.

In these studies, scientists found that after PEMF treatment the blood volume increased, blood oxygen content was boosted, and the pH became more alkaline - a condition regarded as helpful for treating and preventing a number of diseases.[7]

In summary, the positive effects of PEMFs on circulation can be explained by several mechanisms:

- Dilation of blood vessels (Nitric Oxide [NO] mediated vasodilation)

- Formation of new blood vessels through increased secretion of growth hormones FGF-2 / VEGF (neoangiogenesis)

- Reduction of adhesion of platelets

- Reduction of fibrinogen and improvement of fibrinolysis

- Improvement of the ductility of the red blood cells so that they can be transported through capillaries more easily

PEMFs for Fighting Inflammation

Inflammation is an incredibly powerful force within our bodies. In the short term, this process powerfully protects our bodies from injury and infection by rushing blood and immune cells to the site

---

7 Warmke U. Survey of some working mechanisms of pulsating electromagnetic fields PEMF). Bioelectrochem Bioeneg 27(3):317-320,1992.

of an injury and blocking the ability of invading cells to spread throughout the body.

However, when it becomes chronic, these aspects of inflammation actually interfere with the body's ability to heal and function in a healthy way.

The negative effects of chronic inflammation are so common and pervasive that the long-term presence of inflammation markers in the blood are correlated with worse outcomes in almost every disease.

In most people, inflammation markers steadily rise as we get older. Some doctors now believe chronic inflammation to be a major source of the reduced vitality and increased incidence of disease that occur as we age.

A dazzling variety of medical conditions and age-related declines can be treated by reducing inflammation using drugs, diet, and any other method available. For some conditions, health experts recommend that reducing inflammation become a #1 priority to improve and preserve health and to slow down age-related tissue damage.

This is another area where PEMF can help. Through its biochemical effects, PEMF can be part of your healthy inflammation-reduction regimen.

PEMFs for Broken Bones, Including Non-Healing Fractures

A "fracture" is of course a broken bone - breakage in the hard, mineralized tissue created by osteoblasts. "Delayed unions" and "non-unions" are fractured bones that have not yet grown back together into a whole and healed bone.

Sometimes, the body can even "accept" a fractured bone as being normal. In these cases, the body stops sending "grow new bone" messages entirely before healing is complete. In these cases, the fracture may never heal without medical help. Needless to say, broken bones have a significant impact on patients' quality of life, their medical conditions, and their ability to work.[8]

You'll probably remember from our earlier chapter on osteogenic loading that Dr. Julius Wolff determined that it is the bending, or deformation of bones that causes "grow new bone" signals to be released. But you might not know that in 1953, Dr. Iwao Yasuda revealed that bending the long tubular bone is correlated to the development of electric currents, and this instance is defined as piezoelectric phenomenon.

In other words, bones seem to use electromagnetic charges as the medium for the "grow new bone signals" they send in response to osteogenic loading.[9]

Today, scientists know that bone building and bone breakdown are influenced by electrical charge. Bone tends to be broken down under "electropositive" conditions, while new bone tends to be built under "electronegative" conditions.

In fact, it's thought that these electrical conditions are the mechanism by which the body tells its cells whether to build or break down bone. The more we learn about our body's internal signaling systems, the more logical this conclusion becomes: the flow of electrically charged atoms is used to direct countless processes within our bodies.[10]

As we know, PEMF has the power to affect the charge conditions of the body's cells in a non-invasive way. Because electrical charge and magnetism are part of the same unified physical force,

---

8 Victoria G, Petrisor B, Drew B, et al. 2009. Bone stimulation for fracture healing: What's all the fuss? Indian J Orthop 2009; 43:117-120.

9 The classic: Fundamental aspects of fracture treatment by Iwao Yasuda, reprinted from J. Kyoto Med. Soc., 4: 395-406, 1953. Clin Orthop Relat Res 1977 5-8.

10 Schemitsch E, Kuzyk P. The science of electrical stimulation therapy for fracture healing. *Indian Journal of Orthopaedics*. 2009;43(2):127. doi:10.4103/0019-5413.50846.

magnetic fields can be used to move and change electrical potential in a safe and gentle way.

Several clinical studies have shown that devices using electrical currents and magnetic fields can stimulate bone growth and healing, and they can be especially useful in treating bone fractures that have not healed on their own. Many devices have been developed to produce electrical stimulation for promoting the healing of bone fractures.

In 1978, Bassett first applied noninvasive PEMFs to treat delayed union or non-union fractures - fractures where the broken bone has not healed to form a single, unified bone mass as expected. These PEMFs achieved a positive clinical effect,[11] and were approved as a safe and effective method for treating delayed union or non-union fractures by the US Food and Drug Administration (FDA).[12][13]

It's thought that PEMFs stimulate bone growth and healing through a mechanism called inductive coupling.[14] PEMF devices consist of a wire coil through which a current is passed and a pulsed magnetic field is generated. The pulsed magnetic field, in turn, induces a time-varying electrical field within the bone.

This electrical field may mimic the body's natural "build new bone" signals, which may be especially important in cases where the body seems to have "accepted" a non-union, or unhealed fracture, and has stopped sending its own natural signals to the bone to re-grow.

---

11 Bassett CA, Mitchell SN, Norton L, et al. 1978. Repair of non-unions by pulsing electromagnetic fields. Acta Orthop Belg 1978; 44:706-724.

12 Gupta AK, Srivastava KP, Avasthi S. 2009. Pulsed electromagnetic stimulation in nonunion of tibial diaphyseal fractures. Indian J Orthop 2009; 43:156-160.

13 Meskens MW, Stuyck JA, Feys H, et al. 1990. Treatment of nonunion using pulsed electromagnetic fields: a retrospective follow-up study. Acta Orthop Belg 1990; 56:483-488.

14 Assiotis A, Sachinis NP, Chalidis BE. 2012. Pulsed electromagnetic fields for the treatment of tibial delayed unions and nonunions. A prospective clinical study and review of the literature. J Orthop Surg Res 2012; 7:24.

Through the PEMF device, a time-varying electrical field is produced to simulate the normal response of bone cells physiologically to the applied mechanical stress,[15] and the subsequent enhanced growth and remodeling bioeffects on the bone are initiated by the time-varying electrical field.

The secondary electrical field produced by PEMFs in bone is dependent on the characteristics of the applied pulsed magnetic field and the tissue properties. Magnetic fields of 0.1–20 G are usually applied to produce electrical fields, ranging from 1 mV/cm to 100 mV/cm in the bone.[16]

For nearly forty years since their approval by the FDA, gentle and non-invasive PEMFs have been used effectively in clinics as physical therapy to accelerate and finalize the healing process of newly broken bones, and to reactivate the healing process of delayed unions and non-unions.[17][18]

A recent systematic review and meta-analysis of randomized controlled trials showed that PEMFs significantly shortened the time to radiological union - the point where a fracture is no longer detectable on X-ray - for acute fractures that did not require surgery.

PEMF also significantly shortened the healing time of acute fractures of the upper limbs and accelerated the time to clinical union for acute fractures of the central shaft of long bones.[19]

15 Kuzyk PR, Schemitsch EH. 2009. The science of electrical stimulation therapy for fracture healing. Indian J Orthop 2009; 43:127-131

16 Chalidis B, Sachinis N, Assiotis A, et al. 2011. Stimulation of bone formation and fracture healing with pulsed electromagnetic fields: biologic responses and clinical implications. Int J Immunopathol Pharmacol 2011; 24:17-20.

17 Gupta AK, Srivastava KP, Avasthi S. 2009. Pulsed electromagnetic stimulation in nonunion of tibial diaphyseal fractures. Indian J Orthop 2009; 43:156-160.

18 Meskens MW, Stuyck JA, Feys H, et al. 1990. Treatment of nonunion using pulsed electromagnetic fields: a retrospective follow-up study. Acta Orthop Belg 1990; 56:483-488.

19 Hannemann PF, Mommers EH, Schots JP, et al. 2014. The effects of low-intensity pulsed ultrasound and pulsed electromagnetic fields bone growth

Another study that evaluated the effect of PEMFs on 64 patients who needed to have joints in their feet fused together to prevent movement for medical reasons (144 joints) revealed that the use of a PEMF in joint fusion surgeries may increase the rate and speed of radiographic union - or complete healing and fusion - of these joints.[20]

Despite the relative scarcity of well-organized randomized controlled trials, many studies highlight the practical usefulness of PEMFs in treating delayed unions or non-unions of the tibia bone in the leg, with up to 87% of patients with delayed or non-healing fractures recovering after PEMF use.[21][22]

In a broad literature review comparing PEMF treatment of non-unions with surgical therapy, Gossling noted that 81% of reported cases healed with PEMF versus 82% with surgery. PEMFs were shown to be more effective than surgery for healing non-unions breaks complicated by infections (81% versus 69%), and non-unions caused by closed injuries (85% versus 79%).[23]

In addition, a recent double-blind randomized study showed that the use of PEMF for fifth metatarsal fracture non-unions significantly shortened the average time to complete radiographic union. While the control group which did not receive PEMF

stimulation in acute fractures: a systematic review and meta-analysis of randomized controlled trials. Arch Orthop Trauma Surg 2014; 134:1093-1106.

20 Dhawan SK, Conti SF, Towers J, et al. 2004. The effect of pulsed electromagnetic fields on hindfoot arthrodesis: a prospective study. J Foot Ankle Surg 2004; 43:93-96.

21 Bassett CA, Mitchell SN, Gaston SR. 1981. Treatment of ununited tibial diaphyseal fractures with pulsing electromagnetic fields. J Bone Joint Surg Am 1981; 63:511-523.

22 de Haas WG, Watson J, Morrison DM. 1980. Non-invasive treatment of ununited fractures of the tibia using electrical stimulation. J Bone Joint Surg Br 1980; 62-B:465-470.

23 Nelson FR, Brighton CT, Ryaby J, et al. 2003. Use of physical forces in bone healing. J Am Acad Orthop Surg 2003; 11:344-354.

treatment took 14.7 weeks to heal, patients who received PEMF treatment took only 8.9 weeks.

Elevated expression levels of PIGF, BMP-5, and BMP-7 - key cellular signals promoting bone and blood vessel growth - were first detected in non-healing fractures before and after the application of PEMFs.[24]

These studies strikingly support PEMFs as an effective method to accelerate fracture healing and improve outcomes in cases of injury.

PEMFs for Osteoporosis & Bone Density

Osteoporosis is a worldwide health problem. It's increasingly common and can negatively impact quality of life, especially in postmenopausal women.[252627] It is generally defined as a systemic skeletal disease characterized by low bone mineral density (BMD) and compromised bone strength, leading to bone fragility, increased fracture risk, and resulting complications and disability.[282930]

---

24 Zhou W, Yu L, Fan J, et al. 2017. Endogenous Parathyroid Hormone Promotes Fracture Healing by Increasing Expression of BMPR2 through cAMP/PKA/CREB Pathway in Mice. Cell Physiol Biochem 2017; 42:551-563.

25 Pai MV. 2017. Osteoporosis Prevention and Management. J Obstet Gynaecol India 2017; 67:237-242.

26 Golob AL, Laya MB. 2015. Osteoporosis: screening, prevention, and management. Med Clin North Am 2015; 99:587-606.

27 Verbovoy AF, Pashentseva AV, Sharonova LA. 2017. Osteoporosis: Current state of the art. Ter Arkh 2017; 89:90-97.

28 Ensrud KE, Crandall CJ. 2017. Osteoporosis. Ann Intern Med 2017; 167:ITC17-ITC32.

29 Watts NB, Bilezikian JP, Camacho PM, et al. 2010. American Association of Clinical Endocrinologists Medical Guidelines for Clinical Practice for the diagnosis and treatment of postmenopausal osteoporosis. Endocr Pract 2010; 16:S1-37.

30 Eyres KS, Saleh M, Kanis JA. 1996. Effect of pulsed electromagnetic fields on bone formation and bone loss during limb lengthening. Bone 1996; 18:505-509.

In the 1970s, NASA scientists showed that PEMFs can be just as effective as mechanical stimulation at maintaining or improving bone mass. Since then, many clinical studies have achieved positive therapeutic effects for osteoporosis using PEMFs.[31][32][33][34][35][36]

Chronic pain is a common symptom experienced by people with osteoporosis.[37] Degeneration of bone and joints can lead to unpleasant or even debilitating pain that becomes a patient's constant companion. Fortunately, PEMFs can help with this symptom in addition to restoring and preserving bone density.

Bone metabolism is a continual cycle of bone growth and resorption. As we've discussed in earlier chapters, our body is constantly adjusting our bone density based on the amount of bone it "thinks" we need. It consumes bone if we spend time being sedentary, and creates new bone when we send it messages that more bone is needed, such as through osteogenic loading.

These processes are carefully orchestrated by the dynamic relationship between osteoclasts (cells that break down bone),

31 Rubin CT, McLeod KJ, Lanyon LE. 1989. Prevention of osteoporosis by pulsed electromagnetic fields. J Bone Joint Surg Am 1989; 71:411-417.

32 Tabrah F, Hoffmeier M, Bassett CA, et al. 1990. Bone density changes in osteoporosis-prone women exposed to pulsed electromagnetic fields (PEMFs). J Bone Miner Res 1990; 5:437-442.

33 Garland DE, Adkins RH, Matsuno NN, et al. 1999. The effect of pulsed electromagnetic fields on osteoporosis at the knee in individuals with spinal cord injury. J Spinal Cord Med 1999; 22:239-245.

34 Liu H, Liu Y, Yang L, et al. 2014. Curative effects of pulsed electromagnetic fields on postmenopausal osteoporosis. Sheng Wu Yi Xue Gong Cheng Xue Za Zhi 2014; 31:48-52.

35 Wang R, Wu H, Yang Y, et al. 2016. Effects of electromagnetic fields on osteoporosis: A systematic literature review. Electromagn Biol Med 2016; 35:384-390.

36 Weng YX, Gao QY, Shao HWy, et al. 2003. Osteoporosis pain and effectiveness of pulsed electromagnetic fields in treating pain in patients with osteoporosis. Chin J Osteoporos (China)2003; 9:3-17.

37 Hayashi Y. 2007. Bone diseases with Pain. Osteoporosis. Clin Calcium 2007; 17:606-612.

osteoblasts (cells that make more bone) and an array of hormones and other chemical messengers.

The relative levels of these chemical messengers "tell" the cells involved in bone metabolism what to do and determine whether our bone metabolism remains healthy and balanced.

Disturbances to these messaging systems can weaken the skeletal architecture and put one at risk for the development of chronic and debilitating diseases such as osteoporosis.

In osteoporosis, a breakdown of bone mass and the destruction of the microarchitecture of bone tissue increases the risk of fractures. It becomes more common with age and is the most common reason for a broken bone among the elderly.

About 15% of people in their 50s and 70% of people over 80 are affected. Osteoporosis is more common in women than men because hormonal changes occurring during menopause can increase bone loss.

Bones that commonly break include the vertebrae, the bones of the forearm, and the hip. These fractures can be devastating in elderly patients and can threaten mobility or even cause life-threatening complications.

Until a broken bone occurs, there are typically no symptoms of osteoporosis. Bones may weaken to such a degree that a fracture may occur with minor stress, such as from walking, or even spontaneously.

Certain medications increase the rate of bone loss, including some antiseizure medications, chemotherapy, proton pump inhibitors (including some common heartburn medications), selective serotonin reuptake inhibitors (including some common antidepressants), and glucocorticosteroids. Smoking and too little exercise are also risk factors.

Osteoporosis is defined as a bone density of 2.5 standard deviations below that of a healthy young adult. This is typically measured by dual-energy X-ray absorptiometry, also called a DXA or DEXA test.

Efforts to prevent broken bones in those with osteoporosis include proper nutrition and exercise. Exercise, however, must accomplish an osteogenic loading effect, which "tells" the body that more bone density is needed.

Randomized controlled trials have shown that PEMF exposure can relieve chronic pain caused by osteoporosis.[38] In one study of 126 patients, PEMF provided fast and significant pain relief for patients with type I primary osteoporosis, which tends to begin earlier in life than type II osteoporosis which is most common after the age of 70.[39]

One study of twenty women with osteoporosis showed that BMD increased in bones treated using PEMFs.[40]

In another study, which evaluated the effect of PEMFs on knee osteoporosis in patients with spinal cord injury, BMD was also found to increase after treatment. Three months into the study protocol, BMD was increased by 5.1% in the PEMF-treated knees but *declined* by 6.6% in the control knees which were not treated with PEMFs.

Using PEMFs as a noninvasive physical therapy method for osteoporosis avoids the negative effects of pharmacotherapy for oste-oporosis, including the multiple medical side effects, higher cost, and the low persistence of effect after medication treatment is stopped.

More importantly, a randomized, active-controlled clinical trial on postmenopausal osteoporosis (PMO) in Southwest China revealed that PEMFs had the same effect as alendronate, which is the most commonly prescribed medication for treating PMO.[41]

38 Verbovoy AF, Pashentseva AV, Sharonova LA. 2017. Osteoporosis: Current state of the art. Ter Arkh 2017; 89:90-97.

39 Ensrud KE, Crandall CJ. 2017. Osteoporosis. Ann Intern Med 2017; 167:ITC17-ITC32.

40 Fang QQ, Li ZZ, Zhou J, et al. 2016. Low-frequency pulsed electromagnetic fields promotes rat osteoblast differentiation in vitro through cAMP/PKA signal pathway. Nan Fang Yi Ke Da Xue Xue Bao 2016; 36:1508-1513.

41 Liu HF, Yang L, He HC, et al. 2013. Pulsed electromagnetic fields on post-

The safety of PEMFs for treating osteoporosis has also been observed in randomized, placebo-controlled clinical studies.[42] In numerous studies PEMF has demonstrated its positive effects on bone metabolism. PEMFs have been documented to stimulate bone-building osteoblasts and increase calcium uptake and mineralization, both in vitro (in laboratory dishes) and in vivo (inside living bodies).

All of these results suggest that PEMFs are an ideal partner for osteogenic loading in the quest for strong bones, which is why we've made them available at most OsteoStrong facilities.

PEMFs for Pain Management

You might have noticed that many of the conditions discussed so far - osteoporosis, broken bones, and inflammation - come with one very important and unpleasant symptom. All of them can come with chronic pain.

There are many definitions for the term "pain." Internationally recognized is the definition of the International Association for the Study of Pain (IASP):[43]

"Pain is an unpleasant sensory or emotional experience associated with actual or potential tissue damage or described in terms of such injury."

Acute pain is a warning signal that informs the body about

menopausal osteoporosis in Southwest China: a randomized, active-controlled clinical trial. Bioelectromagnetics 2013; 34:323-332.

42 Liu H, Yang L, He H, et al. 2013. The hemorheological safety of pulsed electromagnetic fields in postmenopausal women with osteoporosis in southwest China: a randomized, placebo controlled clinical trial. Clin Hemorheol Microcirc 2013; 55:285-295.

43 Part III: Pain Terms, A Current List with Definitions and Notes on Usage. Classification of Chronic Pain, Second Edition, IASP Task Force on Taxonomy, edited by H. Merskey and N. Bogduk, IASP Press, Seattle, 1994, pp 209-214.

impending or existing damage. So acute pain has an important role to play in helping us stay safe and avoid injury.

However, pain can also occur without cause. Once pain has delivered its helpful message, we'd very much like it to go away.

These chronic pains that persist long after an acute injury, or arise from a chronic health condition, have lost their warning function. They serve no purpose except to impair our quality of life.

Whether acute or chronic, strong or long-lasting, dull or stinging, pain represents an enormous physical and emotional burden for those affected. Pain is not only a pure sensory perception, but also an unpleasant emotional event and a decrease in quality of life.

Pain development follows a classical stimulus-response mechanism. If the body is confronted with a harmful stimulus, so-called nociceptors - sensors of "noxious," or harmful things - are activated.

These pain receptors are very common in the skin, but also in muscles, joints, and in the walls of blood vessels and internal organs.

These nociceptors are widely branched endings of special nerve cells that respond to various pain causes. Harmful events that may cause pain to warn us of tissue damage include chemicals, heat, and trauma such as cuts or bruises. Sometimes internal processes such as infections, immune system reactions, or nerves becoming pinched between bones can also create warning pain signals.

The stronger the stimulus, the greater the number of activated pain receptors and released mediators of inflammation, and thus the strength of the perceived pain increases. But sometimes those receptors can *stay* activated after the threat has passed, or become activated for no reason in conditions such as fibromyalgia.

Relieving Chronic Pain

Pain becomes chronic when it has lost its proper function as a warning and protection signal. Chronic pain is usually defined as pain that persists for more than three months or occurs at intervals over a long period of time. The pain is then considered an independent disease, which cannot be treated by treating a root injury or cause but must instead be treated by itself simply for pain relief.

The causes of chronic pain can include inadequate treatment of acute pain, and many chronic and incurable diseases. The most common forms of chronic pain include back pain, headache, cancer-related pain, and rheumatic pain. With increasing age, the progression of chronic pain increases.

> *"One in five adults in Europe suffer from chronic pain,*
> *25% of whom cannot fully participate in social life,*
> *and this has physical and psychological effects - on*
> *the individual, his or her partner, children, parents*
> *and grandparents, neighbors and many others."*

> - Joop van Griensven, President
> of the European Pain Alliance

For sufferers, the ongoing pain is an enormous burden that severely limits their quality of life. This in turn can lead to further illnesses such as depression.

The good news is, there are many different steps to the transmission and processing of pain. Each of these steps represents an opportunity to interrupt or interfere with the process, thereby reducing the experience of pain.

We'll discuss here some ways in which doctors and scientists can interfere with or reduce the experience of pain, including how PEMFs can help.

Current medical approaches to pain therapy include pharmacological, surgical and physical options. Although many patients can be provided with pain relief in this way, not all of them respond to or are suitable for these options. Pharmacological and surgical therapy approaches also carry risks which are best avoided wherever possible.

The most commonly used painkillers are so-called non-opioid analgesics such as ibuprofen, paracetamol, diclofenac or acetylsalicylic acid. Not only do these have an analgesic effect, they also have anti-inflammatory and antipyretic (anti-fever) effects.

However, their side effect list, especially in higher doses, is long. Long-term use of these compounds can have risks including "refractory pain" (where pain is experienced more severely if the medication is stopped) and bleeding.

For severe pain, drugs of the opiate class are necessary, whose high addiction and abuse potential has been highlighted in recent years. Opiates' effect of depressing nervous system activity can even lead to fatal overdoses, where central nervous system activity is suppressed so much that the brain ceases to send signals to keep the lungs breathing.

For people who are looking for help with pain management, PEMFs are an excellent option. Research has shown that effects of PEMF in modulating pain signals can even mimic the administration of opioids, but without the dangerous side effects.

Magnetic fields affect pain perception in many ways, acting at multiple points within the pain transmission process. These actions are both direct and indirect.

How can laying on a PEMF mat reduce pain? Many people who suffer from chronic pain experience a real improvement after using PEMF. To understand how PEMFs relieve pain, we must first understand how pain is created by nerve signals traveling from the body to the brain.

In the course of moving from the body to the brain, pain signals travel through three different types of nerves:

1. Peripheral nerves, which exist in peripheral body parts such as the arms, legs, face, and organs.

2. Spinal nerves, which travel between the peripheral nerves and the spinal cord that carries signals to the brain.

3. Central nerves in the brain and spine, which connect these distress signals from the peripheral nerves to areas of the brain associated with negative emotions.

Each of these types of nerves contain different types of nerve fibers - cells which operate in different ways to transmit pain. We experience pain from these nerve fibers in different ways: for example, we may withdraw our hands from a hot stove *before* actually feeling pain from the burn, because the first, "rapid" distress call got to our brain before the slower C-fiber signal that tells us about any tissue damage we've sustained from the heat.

PEMFs can affect nerves at each of these three stages of the pain transmission process.

Direct effects of magnetic fields include neuron firing, calcium ion movement, strengthened membrane potentials, increased endorphin levels, nitric oxide and dopamine levels, and nerve regeneration. All of these effects have been seen in nervous systems treated with PEMFs and may be explained by PEMFs' influences on charged particles, and on the several intracellular signaling mechanisms discussed in previous sections.

Indirect benefits of magnetic fields on physiologic function include improved circulation, muscle relaxation, reduced edema, improved tissue oxygen, decreased inflammation, increased healing, release of prostaglandins, and improved cellular metabolism and cell energy levels. These do not act directly on pain nerves, but may reduce pain by improving the underlying injury or disease process.

Several authors have reviewed the experience of the medical communities with pulsed electromagnetic therapy (PEMF) in Eastern Europe[44] and the West.[45] EMFs have been used extensively in many conditions and medical disciplines. They have been most effective in treating rheumatic and musculoskeletal disorders.

Although PEMFs have been proven to be a powerful tool, they should always be considered in combination with other therapeutic procedures. As we've stated regarding other medical conditions, PEMFs should help, but patients should always seek professional diagnosis and follow doctors' orders rather than taking it upon themselves to seek treatment without professional medical help.

Pain-related conditions where PEMFs have shown preclinical (laboratory animal studies) or clinical (studies in human patients) effectiveness include:

- Success in reducing chronic lower back pain,[4647] from causes including herniated lumbar discs, spondylosis, radiculopathy,[48] sciatica, arthritis, and osteochondrosis.[49]

44 Jerabek, J and Pawluk, W. Magnetic therapy in Eastern Europe: a review of 30 years of research. Publ. Advanced Magnetic Research of the Delaware Valley, Chicago, 1996.

45 Trock DH. Electromagnetic fields and magnets. Investigational treatment for musculoskeletal disorders. Rheum Dis Clin North Am 2000 Feb;26(1):51-62, viii.

46 Preszler, RR. A non-invasive complementary method of reducing chronic muscular low back pain using permanent magnetic therapy. A Thesis For the degree of Masters in Physician Assistant Studies University of Nebraska School of Medicine, Physician Assistant Program, Lincoln, Nebraska, 2000.

47 Rauscher E, Van Bise W. L. Pulsed magnetic field treatment of chronic back pain. Bioelectromagnetics Society, 23rd Annual Meeting, St. Paul, MN, June,2001.

48 Thuile C, Walzl M. Evaluation of electromagnetic fields in the treatment of pain in patients with lumbar radiculopathy or the whiplash syndrome. NeuroRehabilitation 2002; 17: 63-67.

49 Mitbreit IM, Savchenko AG, et al. Low-frequency magnetic field in the complex treatment of patients with lumbar osteochondrosis. Ortop Travmatol Protez (10):24-27, 1986.

- Success in reducing headache,[50] migraine,[51] neck,[52] shoulder and arm pain.[53]

- Success in reducing chronic musculoskeletal pain.[545556]

- Success in modulating neurologic pain signal processing.[57]

- Success in decreasing the density of brain opiate receptors and pain perception[5859] and increasing pain threshold.[60]

50 Prusinski A, Wielka J, Durko A. Pulsating electromagnetic field in the therapy of headache. J Bioelectr 7(1):127-128 Second Symposium on Magnetotherapy, Szekesfehervar, Hungary, May, 1987.

51 Sherman, R. A.; Acosta, N. M.; Robson, L. Treatment of migraine with pulsing electromagnetic fields: a double-blind, placebo-controlled study. Headache 39(8):567-575, 1999.

52 Foley-Nolan, D.; Barry, C.; Coughlan, R. J.; O'Connor, P.; Roden, D. Pulsed high frequency (27 mhz) electromagnetic therapy for persistent neck pain. A double blind, placebo-controlled study of 20 patients. Orthopedics 13(4):445-451, 1990.

53 Kjellman GV, Skargren EI, Oberg BE. A critical analysis of randomised clinical trials on neck pain and treatment efficacy. A review of the literature. Scand J Rehabil Med 31(3):139-152, 1999.

54 Stewart DJ, Stewart JE. Acta Med Hung 1989;46(4):323-37. The destabilization of an abnormal physiological balanced situation, chronic musculoskeletal pain, utilizing magnetic biological device.

55 Kobinger W, Fischer G, et al. Using Magnetic Fields to Increase Flexibility and Reduce Pain with Respect to Ailments of the Ambulatory Apparatus. 26th Conference of the Austrian Society for Internal Medicine. July 1995.

56 Pujol J, Pascual Leone A, et al. The effect of repetitive magnetic stimulation on localized musculoskeletal pain. Neuroreport 9(8):1745-1748, 1998.

57 Thomas AW, Prato FS. Magnetic field based pain therapeutics and diagnostics. Bioelectromagnetics Society, 24th Annual Meeting, Quebec City, PQ, Canada, June, 2002

58 Ghione S, Luschi P, et al. Electromagnetic fields and nociception: physiological and clinical responses. Forum on Future European Research on Mobile Communications and Health, Bordeaux, France, April, 1999.

59 Sartucci F, Bonfiglio L, et al. Changes in pain perception and pain-related somatosensory evoked potentials in humans produced by exposure to oscillating magnetic fields. Brain Res 769(2):362-366, 1997.

60 Fleming, JL, Persinger, MA, et al. Magnetic pulses elevate nociceptive

- Success in reducing pain in toothache[61] and stomatology.[62]

- Success in improving healing of bone fractures.[63]

- Success in reducing edema and swelling resulting from illness or injury.[64]

- Success in improving osteoarthritis[6566]

- Success in improving post-herpetic neuralgia.[67]

- Success in improving neuropathic pain.[68]

- Success in improving coxarthrosis.[69]

- Success in improving diabetic neuropathy.[70]

thresholds: comparisons with opiate receptor compounds in normal and sei-zure-induced brain-damaged rats. Electro Magnetobiol 13(1):67-75, 1994.

61 Hutchinson D, Witt S, Fairpo CG. Pulsed electromagnetic energy therapy in third molar surgery. Oral Surg Oral Med Oral Pathol, 46(6):748-754, 1978.

62 Tesic D, Djuric M, et al. PEMF aided pain reduction in stomatology. Bioelectromagnetics Society, 21st Annual Meeting, Long Beach, CA, Abstract, June, 1999.

63 Schroter M. Conservative Treatment of 240 Patients with Magnetic Field Therapy. Medizinisch- Orthopadische Technik. March/April 1976 (2):78.

64 Markov MS, Pilla A. A. Electromagnetic field stimulation of soft tissue: pulsed radiofrequency treatment of post-operative pain and edema. Wounds 7(4):143-151, 1995.

65 Jacobson JL, Gorman R, Yamanashi WS, et al. Low-amplitude, extremely low frequency magnetic fields for the treatment of osteoarthritic knees: a double-blind clinical study. Altern Ther Health Med 7(5):54-60, 62-64, 66-69, 2001.

66 Pawluk W, Turk Z, et al. Treatment of osteoarthritis with a new broadband PEMF signal. Bioelectromagnetics Society, 24th Annual Meeting, Quebec City, QC, Canada, June,2002.

67 Kusaka C, Seto A, et al. Pulse magnetic treatment and whole-body, alternating current magnetic treatment for post-herpetic neuralgia. J Jpn Biomagnetism Bioelectromagnetics Soc 8(2):29-38, 1995.

68 Munglani R. The longer term effect of pulsed radiofrequency for neuropathic pain. Pain 80(1-2):437-439, 1999.

69 Rehacek J, Straub J, Benova H. The effect of magnetic fields on coxar-throses. Fysiatr Revmatol Vestn 60(2):66-68, 1982.

70 Cieslar G, Sieron A, Radelli J. The estimation of therapeutic effect of vari-

More research is needed to further develop the mechanisms and optimal treatment parameters for the use of PEMFs for pain. But what we do know so far is that PEMFs of various kinds, strengths, and frequencies have been found to have good results in a wide array of painful conditions.

There is little risk to PEMF treatment when compared to the side effects and invasiveness of other therapies, making PEMF an appealing option for most chronic pain patients.

PEMFs for Reducing Edema

Edema is swelling caused by excess fluid in your tissues. It most often occurs due to an imbalance of charged particles, called ions, in your body. These ion imbalances can be caused by a wide variety of conditions, including hormonal conditions, kidney problems, injury, and poor nutrition.

The consequences of edema can be serious, including impaired circulation of oxygen, nutrients, and waste products, and potentially even cell death and tearing of the surrounding tissues.

PEMF therapy acts directly on the sodium-potassium pump in the cell membrane to restore the balance of charged particles and fluids. Improving the circulation of blood also helps to remove excess fluid and ions and prevent further accumulation of fluid. Anti-edema effects are rapid after using PEMFs.[71]

PEMFs not only improve blood circulation, but also have a positive effect on lymphatic vessels - a type of vessel that carries non-blood fluid rich in immune cells and cellular waste products to the kidneys through the lymphatic system.

PEMF stimulates lymphatic drainage and reduces lymphoe-

---

able magnetic fields in patients with diabetic neuropathy including vibratory sensibility. Balneol Pol, 1995, 37(1): 23-27.
71 Jerabek J, Pawluk W. Magnetic therapy in Eastern Europe: a review of 30 years of research. Publ Advanced Magnetic Research of the Delaware Valley, Chicago, 1996.

dema - swelling due to lymphatic buildup. This benefit improves the circulation of immune cells around the body, and the elimination of waste.

PEMF and OsteoStrong

Michael Faraday stated Faraday's Law in 1831, which established that a time-varying electrical current creates a magnetic field that can in turn induce an electric field. His law went on to state that this field can create a secondary current within a nearby conducting medium.

In 1982, working from Columbia University School of Medicine, Dr. Andrew Bassett published a series of four articles on the positive effects of pulsating electromagnetic fields for non-healing bone fracture in three well-known North American medical journals. As a result of Bassett's work, the FDA approved the sawtooth waveform in 1979 for the treatment of non-union bone fractures and aid in spinal fusion operations.

Almost fifty years after Basset reported his findings, OsteoStrong began using their first PEMF device to hack the therapeutic benefits of the osteogenic loading process.

Because one major benefit of PEMF is stimulating bone growth, PEMF is a natural partner for OsteoStrong's bone density technology. Inducing bone growth through osteogenic loading and adding the benefits of PEMF just made sense.

The device did not need to be in direct contact with the tissues of the body because the electric field produces a magnetic field, which permeates the air - and any body parts that may happen to be nearby. This PEMF produces a current in the conductive tissues, including bone tissues which read its small electrical currents as growth signals.

This provided OsteoStrong members with a seamless therapeutic modality that integrated OsteoStrong's mission of promoting skeletal strength, along with the additional health benefits of PEMF therapy.

Like all good biohacks, this regimen was quick, easy, and did not require expending effort or enduring pain to achieve astounding results.

OsteoStrong's founder partnered with Swiss Bionic Solutions in their bid to deliver these benefits to people everywhere.

Swiss Bionic Solutions Manufacturing Standards

We at OsteoStrong selected the device manufactured by Swiss Bionic to bring PEMF into our facilities. Our decision came after a long process and thorough vetting to ensure that we found the best manufacturer of PEMFs on the market to meet our member's needs.

A globally organized company with Swiss origin, Swiss Bionic Solutions develops and distributes innovative health and wellness products worldwide in the fields of complementary and alternative medicine. In recent years, Swiss Bionic Solutions has specialized particularly in "bionic solutions."

"Bionics" is the science of discovering "inventions of active nature" which have effects on living tissues. The low-energy frequencies and intensities in the Earth's geomagnetic field serve as a natural "bionic" model which can be mimicked by human technology.

Swiss Bionic Solutions' core iMRS technology is used in more home-use systems than any other PEMF system in the world. The iMRS offers the same uncompromising German-engineered quality and reliability and sets a new industry standard for in-home efficacy, aesthetic, ergonomic comfort and user-friendliness.

PEMF devices for home use have been on the market for nearly two decades. Swiss Bionic Solutions is the only PEMF company world-wide with its own research & development, engineering, and manufacturing divisions.

This track record began with iMRS-series technology. The more than 3.65 billion applications of this technology world-wide have solidified Swiss Bionic Solutions' standing as the leader in pulsed electromagnetic field devices.

As a manufacturer of PEMF devices, Swiss Bionic Solutions is certified through the international standards of the Medical Device Single Audit Program (MDSAP) for the design and development, manufacturing, distribution and service of pulsed electromagnetic field therapy devices.

Swiss Bionic Solutions' PEMF devices are available to consumers around the world without a prescription.

As we'll soon see, PEMF isn't the only surprising use of electromagnetic energy for your health.

CHAPTER 5

Hack Your Mitochondria with Light Therapy
Scott Nelson
Co-Founder, Joovv

LIGHT THERAPY - also known as "photobiomodulation" or "red light therapy" - is a powerful, non-invasive treatment that can improve our cells' abilities to produce energy and heal. In light therapy, a device delivers concentrated wavelengths of light to the skin and underlying tissues.

Light therapy has become a popular treatment in recent years due to evidence that it enhances the health of skin, muscles, joints, the skeletal system, improves sleep quality, and even fights pain & inflammation.

But light isn't usually included in the story when we're taught about the benefits of nutrition, exercise, or overall healthy lifestyle. Conventional wisdom doesn't say anything about the effects of the light our bodies receive on our health.

So how in the world does this work? Clinical studies show benefits from red light therapy through recently discovered pathways in the mitochondria - those all-important creators of energy and health that live within our cells.

Modern Life Has a Light Problem

Most people don't realize it, but America has a light problem. In our modern world, many people are now exposed to more artificial light than natural light. It's so extreme that surveys are finding the average American spends over 90% of their time indoors.

This is a serious health risk. When inventing artificial light, our ancestors didn't stop to wonder if these artificial light sources would have the healthiest wavelengths our bodies need, or if some wavelengths of light might actually be bad for us. But we now know that our bodies need natural light every day, just like we need water and food.

This has not been as easy for scientists to discover, because most people received sufficient natural light in their daily lives for most of human history. There was never danger of an extended "sun famine," and no region of the world where sun doesn't shine for about half of the hours in a year.

As a result, scientists took natural light for granted. They assumed it was not important to our health, and attributed health problems that arose with the movement of modern life indoors solely to other factors such as diet and physical activity.

But recent science has revealed that our mitochondria are actually light-sensitive. That is, the biochemical processes which produce our cells' energy respond to, and can be altered by light.

Mitochondria are the "engines" of the cell. They turn food and oxygen into biochemical energy, allowing our bodies to run. By turning oxygen and food into the energy carrier molecule adenosine triphosphate (ATP), our mitochondria allow us to move, think, and stay alive. Mitochondrial efficiency is key to the benefits of PEMF treatment associated with improved circulation and oxygen supply to our cells.

It turns out that, in addition to food and oxygen, mitochondria can also turn sunlight into energy. The more photons of natural light we provide to our mitochondria, the more efficiently they can produce the energy that allows our cells to stay alive and heal us after injuries.

This finding shouldn't be shocking, because the chloroplasts of plants - which harvest sunlight and turn it into fuel - are in many ways similar to our own mitochondria. They use similar mechanisms to produce energy-carrying molecules. But since humans don't immediately die from lack of sunlight, scientists had assumed that our mitochondria couldn't use this as an energy source at all.

Scientists aren't yet entirely sure what biomolecular mechanisms our own mitochondria use to benefit from light. But they now know that the type and amount of light we get affects how much energy our mitochondria produce for us. They know that healthy light speeds healing - and that most people in the modern world today aren't getting enough.

Things like oxidative stress and inflammation slow us down in part because they "gunk up" this basic cellular process of energy production. Aging and poor diet can cause our mitochondria to become damaged and inefficient, resulting in lower energy levels and more toxic waste products.[72]

The opposite happens when our bodies are exposed to red and near-infrared light wavelengths. These wavelengths have the ability to stimulate efficient energy production at the cellular level.

A chronic deficiency of natural light can have a profound negative impact on the body, especially on our sleep, mental health, and energy levels. To make matters worse, it's not just that people don't get enough natural light: it's that they're also getting way too much artificial blue light.

---

72 Klepeis N., Nelson W., Ott W., Robinson J., Tsang A., Switzer P., Behar J., Hern S., Engelmann W. "The National Human Activity Pattern Survey (NHAPS): a resource for assessing exposure to environmental pollutants". Journal of Exposure Analysis and Environmental Epidemiology 2001;11, 231-252.

The Sun produces very little blue light - that's why it looks yellow, which is a combination of red and green light wavelengths.

Our cell phones, tablets, televisions, and computer screens are extremely bright, and contain substantially more blue light than daytime sun. They can be difficult to escape these days, and too much blue light, especially after dark, is a primary reason so many people struggle with sleep. This artificial blue light from screens and bulbs effectively "tells" our cells that it's a bright daytime afternoon, even long after the Sun has set.

Unfortunately, most people who aren't getting enough natural light can't just add 20 hours per week spent outdoors to their busy schedules. People have jobs, commutes, school, kids and parents, and more responsibilities of modern life.

In other words, our modern lifestyles encourage - or even require - being indoors most of the time. Lack of light is often not a personal choice, but a negative feature built into our regular routine, which for many people can't be easily changed.

Even as recently as the nineteenth century, most humans worked in farming or other forms of outdoor labor. Only the Industrial Revolution allowed - and then required - humans to work indoors, with machines, instead of working outdoors with natural materials.

For countless generations, human biology developed around an abundance of natural light. Our routines and technology have radically changed in the last fifty years, but our biology has not. Humans, like all animals, still need natural light to be healthy and make energy.

Natural light is necessary every day to sleep well, heal, and stay in shape. We'll explore the clinical evidence for this need - and how we can use our cells' light-based mechanisms to biohack our healing and our lifestyles - later in this chapter.

What Is Light Therapy?

It's difficult to change our schedules to increase natural light exposure, or reduce blue light exposure in the modern world we live in. While some apps for phones and computers offer to reduce the blue light output of these devices after a certain time of day, lightbulbs do not come with the same technology.

But with light therapy, we can get more of that important exposure to natural light, even if we don't have extra time to be outside. A high-quality light therapy device delivers hours' worth of concentrated healthy wavelengths of light in just a few minutes, and this can be done indoors.

Light therapy was once limited to a few luxury spas and salons, so most people did not have access to this powerful technology. This has been true for decades, despite the fact that medical researchers have published over 1,000 peer-reviewed studies analyzing the positive effects of red and near-infrared light on various medical conditions and on overall health.

Now that light therapy is available for in-home use, and more widely available from practitioners, it's become one of the most popular treatments for skin, fitness, athletics, pain relief, healing, inflammation, and sleep.

The health benefits of light therapy can be far-reaching. Yet the treatments themselves are quite simple, and easy to do in your home. With a medical-grade device, all you really have to do is sit or stand in bright red light for about 10 minutes per day to absorb similar levels of healthy red light to what you would encounter if you spent much of your day outdoors.

OsteoStrong has partnered with Joovv, the leading consumer light therapy brand, to offer full-body red and near infrared light treatments in OsteoStrong clinics.

You will also find Joovv devices being used by professional estheticians & dermatologists for skin care, by trainers and professional athletes for athletic training and recovery, and by a wide range of natural health experts & practitioners.

How Does Light Therapy Work?

Joovv devices use medical-grade light emitting diodes (LEDs) to deliver natural light to your body. When you stand in front of a Joovv device for a treatment, your cells absorb the natural light and your mitochondria become stimulated.

Photomedicine scientists have found that natural light treatments have effects like reducing oxidative stress and increasing circulation, allowing your cells to produce energy more efficiently.

Like water and nutrients from food, our bodies need consistent natural light to make energy. In particular, our cells need all three (water, food, and light) during the core cellular respiration process.

Cellular respiration is a complex biological process that takes place in almost every cell in our body, all the time. In short, a light therapy device works by improving your cellular environment, so you can make more core energy to power and heal yourself every day.

Here are some of the specific benefits which are most well-documented from light therapy.

Eight Big Health Benefits of Light Therapy

Since NASA first started testing red light therapy's potential in the early 1990s, research teams and doctors around the world have discovered more and more possibilities for treating people with natural light. Thousands of studies and trials have been performed on the effectiveness of light therapy, and many more are currently underway.

Clinical research has shown how simple, natural light treatments can have major, positive impacts on your health and fitness. To illustrate the power and possibilities of light therapy, let's take a look at eight of the most well-documented health benefits of natural light treatments, as shown by peer-reviewed clinical research.

For each benefit of light therapy, we'll include an example of a well-known professional who uses Joovv's red light therapy devices and has seen the benefits in their own health and performance.

Quality Sleep with Light Therapy

When you combine a huge lack of natural light in our daily lives with the omnipresence of smartphone, tablet, and computer screens, you get a recipe for poor sleep.

Sleep deprivation causes us to be less alert, have poorer memory retention, and can affect our moods. We're less productive, slower learners, and more likely to make poor decisions when we're tired. Chronic sleep problems can contribute to everything from weight gain to increased inflammation and impaired brain function.

One of the main reasons why many of us sleep so poorly is that our internal clocks, or circadian rhythms, are extremely sensitive to light. Under natural conditions, the relative amounts of blue and red light we experience "tell" our brains when to release sleep hormones, and when to keep us awake.

Our brains and bodies are made to be awake at night and sleep during the day. Everyone knows that. But you might not know that your body actually has light-detecting proteins which promote sleep when the sun's light starts to turn red in the early evening, and promote waking when large amounts of blue light are present, such as in the late morning and early afternoon.

When you look at a bright screen, your body and brain get the "message" that it's time to be alert and awake. In nature, that much blue light means that the sun is nowhere near setting, and you've got a long day ahead of you.

People love binge-watching shows and videos, and often catch a few episodes in bed before they doze off. This can cause confusion within your body. "We're tired, let's sleep" signals can conflict with the "but it's only 10am" signals coming from the blue light your computer or television screen emits.

Watching bright media in a dark room after the sun is down is just about the worst thing you can do for your sleep. You might as well chug an energy drink before you hit the pillow.

This is why so many people are tired all day, yet toss and turn at night when they'd give anything just to get some shut eye. This miscommunication actually encourages your brain to make less of the natural sleep-inducing hormone called melatonin.[73]

Yet many of us do this every night, and we may not find it easy to stop. How can we restore deep, healthy sleep and make the process easy for ourselves?

Natural red and near-infrared light has a lower color temperature than sunlight. It's more similar to the natural light that reaches our eyes around sunrise and sunset - good times to sleep - than the light that reaches them in the late morning or afternoon. These wavelengths are essentially the opposite of the blue light emitted by our screens: instead of telling our body to wake up, red light tells our body it's time to rest.

Research shows that light therapy actually helps people to get more and better sleep, and also helps them produce more of their own natural melatonin.[74]

Sleep studies over the last decade have shown that people treated with red and near infrared light have better sleep outcomes - even people with debilitating sleep disorders.

73 Hatori M., Gronfier C., Van Gelder R., Bernstein P., Carreras J., Panda S., Mark F., Silney D., Hunt C., Hirota T., Furukawa T., Tsubota K. "Global rise of potential health hazards caused by blue light-induced circadian disruption in modern aging societies". NPJ Aging Mech Dis. 2017; 3:9. doi: 10.1038/s41514-017-001-2.
74 Morita T., Tokura H. "Effects of lights of different color temperature on the nocturnal changes in core temperature and melatonin in humans" Journal of Physiological Anthropology. 1996, September; 15(5):243-246.

In one 2018 study, researchers determined that people with serious migraines were able to both reduce the pain and intensity of their headaches with light therapy. Red light therapy was found to be the only treatment tested that helped patients with their sleeping problems as well as their headache symptoms.[75]

Another recent study looked at red light therapy and sleep quality among a group of elite women basketball players. Participants in the study received 14 to 30 minute light therapy sessions once a night for two weeks. With these short but consistent treatment sessions, these athletes saw improved sleep, and researchers found red light therapy to be a nonpharmacologic and noninvasive option for sleep disorder treatment.[76]

Dave Asprey, founder and CEO of Bulletproof, is an influential author and entrepreneur who's written extensively about sleep quality. Mr. Asprey believes sleep is the single most important ingredient to general health and well-being, so he uses a full-body Joovv to regulate his melatonin and light intake.

Mr. Asprey only stays with techniques that work. He says that the results of using Joovv to improve his sleep have been significant. OsteoStrong clients who use the Joovv red light therapy devices available at several OsteoStrong locations say the same.

Light Therapy for Skeletal System Strength

OsteoStrong's founder partnered with Joovv because he wanted to give clients every biohacking advantage possible. It was a natural

---

75 Loeb LM, Amorim RP, et al. "Botulinum toxin A (BT-A) versus low-level laser therapy (LLLT) in chronic migraine treatment: a comparison." Arquivos de neuro-psiquiatria. 2018 Oct;76(10):663-667.
76 Zhao J., Tian Y., Nie J., Xu J., Liu D. "Red light and the sleep quality and endurance performance of Chinese female basketball players" Journal of Athletic Training. 2012, November-December; 47(6):673-678. doi: 10.4085/1062-47.6.08.

partnership for another reason: among red light therapy's benefits is improved skeletal strength and healing.

Light therapy is commonly used for benefits like skin and muscle recovery, but research shows that near-infrared light can penetrate deep into tissues and bone, with well-documented healing and pain relief effects.

One big reason is for this benefit is collagen production. Collagen is one of the most plentiful proteins in the body, forming a key ingredient in skin, muscle, and bone alike.

In study after study, researchers have found higher natural collagen levels in patients treated with red light, and especially with near infrared-light which achieves deep tissue penetration. The results are better than those seen by scientists studying the use of collagen supplements to improve bone, muscle, and skin strength and healing.

And scientists know why: a great deal of collagen from supplements and the food we eat is broken down by the digestive tract before it can be absorbed into our bodies. But when our mitochondria produce more energy, our bodies can produce more of their own natural collagen in our skin, muscle, and bone cells right where it is needed. The result is stronger and healthier skin, bones, muscles, and joints.

A clinical trial in 2014 enrolled fifty people with closed fractures in their wrist or hand. Some received light therapy treatments at the source of the injury, while others only received a placebo treatment for their fractures.

The results were clear: the people treated with light therapy showed significant improvements in their bone injury, while the placebo group did not. Improvements in the light therapy group included less acute pain from the injury, improved grip strength and wrist function, and X-ray images clearly demonstrating structural improvements in the therapy group versus the placebo.[77]

This is just the kind of natural skeletal system treatment we're so excited to offer at OsteoStrong locations worldwide.

Tony Robbins, a promoter of OsteoStrong, and his wife, Sage are both long-time users of Joovv red light therapy.

Light Therapy for Reducing Inflammation

As we've mentioned earlier in this book, inflammation is a major enemy of good health. While it helps to prevent further damage and begin healing during the first stages of injury repair, chronic inflammation can prevent growth and healing from occurring. Chronic inflammation is one common sign of aging, and is thought to be a major cause of age-related health declines.

Inflammation, and the pain and reduced ability to function that it causes, are among the most common medical problems in the United States. Many anti-inflammatory medications are available, but the most widely used NSAID class of drugs has a mixed record of success and failure. Most doctors discourage long-term use of NSAIDs by their patients because of side effects that can become dangerous and uncomfortable over time.

Reducing inflammation is one major benefit of red light therapy. Natural light treatments increase blood flow to damaged tissues, and encourage healing and recovery.[78]

One benefit of light therapy that has found a home in both science and Hollywood is the treatment of muscle pain and inflammation following workouts. Natural light treats muscle soreness

---

77 Chang WD, Wu JH, et al. Therapeutic outcomes of low-level laser therapy for closed bone fracture in the human wrist and hand. Photomedicine and Laser Surgery. 2014 April.

78 Michael R. Hamblin. "Mechanisms and applications of the anti-inflammatory effects of photobiomodulation." AIMS Biophys. 2017; 4(3): 337–361.

and exercise-related inflammation and pain, with strong results after even the most demanding training sessions.[79]

A 2014 trial assessed the benefits of red light therapy administered to healthy young men before they went through "damaging resistance training exercise."

Men in the light therapy group showed far less muscle strength loss, soreness, and range of motion impairment after the workout than those who did the same exercises without light treatments. These results were clinically significant, and the differences were demonstrated to last up to 4 days after a workout.[80]

In other words, even a single light therapy treatment before a physically demanding event can have a major impact on soreness and pain levels days later.

Jorge Cruise is one of the best personal trainers in California, with a long list of big-name Hollywood clients who need to stay in shape. When asked about barriers to getting in the gym for workouts every day, Jorge says that inflammation is what holds most of his clients back. Like anyone else, movie stars miss workouts because of soreness and pain.

Even in celebrities who need to keep fit for their movie roles, inflammation can restrict movement and lead to suboptimal workouts. To combat inflammation and help his clients stick to their workout routines, Jorge started recommending Joovv red light therapy, which he also uses himself.

Jorge reports that this addition has been a game-changer, and

79 Ferraresi C, Bertucci D, Schiavinato J, et al. "Effects of Light-Emitting Diode Therapy on Muscle Hypertrophy, Gene Expression, Performance, Damage, and Delayed-Onset Muscle Soreness: Case-control Study with a Pair of Identical Twins." Am J Phys Med Rehabil. 2016 Oct;95(10):746-57
80 Borges LS, et al. Light-emitting diode phototherapy improves muscle recovery after a damaging exercise. Lasers in Medical Science. 2014 May;29(3):1139-44.

that there are far fewer inflammation-related excuses in his ear now that he's got his clients using Joovv devices in their homes each day. The inflammation that comes with hard work *can* be treated. Light therapy treatments are helping people reduce the strain and pain, so they can stay active and fit.

That goes both for Hollywood stars like Jorge Cruise's clients, and for everyday people who come into OsteoStrong centers looking for relief from inflammation and pain.

Light Therapy For Joint Pain Relief

Over 50 million Americans struggle with forms of arthritis, and millions more have to deal with painful joints from other causes.

Dr. Sarah Ballantyne is a biophysicist, and founder of The Paleo Mom website which breaks down health, fitness, and diet research into actionable items for busy people trying to get healthier.

Dr. Ballantyne speaks directly to women and moms experiencing health problems, because she's one of them. In addition to juggling a family, daily workouts, and a growing business, Dr. Ballantyne was held back for years by persistently painful joints and fibromyalgia.

Fibromyalgia is a condition in which overactive nerves create extreme sensitivity and constant pain throughout the body for no clear reason. This condition has so far proven difficult for doctors to treat, since it does not stem from a specific injury or infectious process. Instead, it seems to lie in how the brain and nerves across the body process daily sensations. In many cases, fibromyalgia cannot be resolved with pharmaceutical options.

Dr. Ballantyne had little success reducing the joint pain she experienced from fibromyalgia - until she tried red light therapy.

According to Dr. Ballantyne, after beginning a regimen of red light therapy her joint pain went away almost entirely for the first time in many years. After nearly two years of daily Joovv use, she says it has not come back, even after demanding Crossfit workouts.

The joint pain benefits Dr. Ballantyne and her readers have found in red light therapy are backed by a large body of clinical research. The biggest benefits can be found in people suffering from rheumatoid arthritis. In those cases, clinical trials have shown that red light therapy can reduce participants' pain by a staggering seventy percent!

Red light therapy has also been found to reduce morning stiffness in trial participants, while improving hand flexibility. It has been used to reduce joint pain in knees and spines, in addition to wrists.[81]

Like Jorge Cruise and his clients, Dr. Ballantyne is using red light therapy to minimize pain and improve function in some of the most painful and essential joints, like the wrists and knees we depend on every day for movement and function.

Improved Training and Performance with Light Therapy

In the last few years, full-body red light therapy systems have started popping up in the locker rooms and training facilities of professional sports teams and athletes.

It's not hard to see why, as study after study has been published in the last decade showing that short natural light treatments can supercharge athletic performance and speed up the crucial muscle recovery phase after training.

This makes sense, given what we know about the role of mitochondria in muscle strength and stamina. If our endurance depends on the mitochondria's ability to produce ATP, anything which can improve the energy output of their "engines" is bound to help.

Clinical research conducted on athletes over the past decade

---

81 Brosseau L, Welch V, et al. Low level laser therapy for osteoarthritis and rheumatoid arthritis: a meta-analysis. The Journal of Rheumatology. Aug 2000; 27(8): 1961-9.

has found that exercise and training plus light therapy is more effective than just exercise and training. Even short, irregular light therapy treatments resulted in increased speed, strength, endurance, and muscle growth in both pro athletes and regular people with average fitness. Regular, consistent light therapy shows even better results.[828384]

Dr. Troy Van Biezen is one of the leading trainers of the PGA, the Professional Golf Association. He works with some of the best players in the world, like Tiger Woods, Jordan Spieth, and other major tournament winners.

Dr. Van Biezen shares that the training room at the world-famous Masters Tournament at Augusta National has a new nickname: now, they call it "the red room."

That's because so many players use Joovv red light therapy devices before and after their rounds to treat their joint pain and inflammation, boost their energy and athleticism, and help them recover after the 18th hole. Joov's focus on supplying the healthy red light found naturally in sunlight has turned the walls of this locker room ruby-red while the machine is in use.

Dr. Van Biezen says just about everyone on the PGA is now using light therapy to help them manage a life on the road and playing tournaments in different cities every week. Even beyond

---

82 Dellagrana RA, Rossato M, et al. Photobiomodulation Therapy on Physiological and Performance Parameters During Running Tests: Dose-Response Effects. Journal of Strength and Conditioning Research. 2018 Oct;32(10):2807-2815.

83 Miranda EF, Tomazoni SS, et al. When is the best moment to apply photobiomodulation therapy (PBMT) when associated to a treadmill endurance-training program? A randomized, triple-blinded, placebo-controlled clinical trial. Lasers in Med Science. 2018 May;33(4):719-727.

84 Vanin AA, et al. What is the best moment to apply phototherapy when associated to a strength training program? A randomized, double-blinded, placebo-controlled trial : Phototherapy in association to strength training. Lasers in Medical Science. 2016 Nov;31(8):1555-1564.

boosting muscle performance, this lifestyle also makes sleep and chronic pain difficult to control - which Joovv can help with, too.

And it's not just golfers. Light therapy has become a go-to training and recovery modality for star NFL players like Keenan Allen with the Chargers and DeMarcus Lawrence with the Cowboys. Light therapy is popular with global athletes competing for gold medals, such as the reigning women's balance beam gold medalist Sanne Wevers, a Dutch gymnast who uses her Joovv to recover from soreness and strain after workouts.

With everything on the line in the PGA, NFL, and other professional sports leagues, the best athletes and trainers are trusting light therapy for a natural competitive edge, with clear results.

These world-famous sports stars wouldn't be using light therapy along with their more traditional workout routines if it didn't produce astounding results on the field and course.

Healthy, Rejuvenated Skin with Red Light

The light therapy benefit that has received the most mainstream attention is probably rejuvenated skin.

The study of red light therapy as a skin treatment began in the hospital setting, with doctors seeking ways to improve outcomes in cases of serious skin injury.

People with wounds, burns, scars, and surgical incisions showed faster and better healing outcomes, with less pain and inflammation along the way when treated with red light therapy. This has even been true for people with serious second and third degree burns. Today, scientists think this effect may be due to the energy-boosting and growth-promoting properties of red light for the skin it touches.

With the cosmetics industry constantly in a race to erase scars and blemishes and provide younger-looking skin to healthy patients, the success of red light therapy in the clinical setting was sure to get their attention.

Back in the dark ages of light therapy, when you could only find it in spas and salons, it was considered a major luxury skin treatment. Its cutting-edge science was restricted to businesses that could pay ten thousand dollars or more and house a bulky machine. The benefits of red-light therapy haven't changed. But now anyone can experience the benefits with smaller, portable machines in their homes, or in a clinic like OsteoStrong.

We've already mentioned how light therapy boosts the production of collagen, which is the foundation of strong and healthy muscles and bones. But the cosmetically minded might also recognize that collagen is the protein found in young, glowing skin. Declining collagen production with age is a major reason for the appearance of wrinkles and sagging skin.

Numerous trials have shown that light therapy treatments improve collagen density in skin, resulting in a big improvement in complexion. The natural anti-inflammatory effect of light therapy also plays a big role in decreasing inflammation-related redness, blemishes, and skin conditions.[858687]

Reduced inflammation and higher collagen density is a natural one-two punch for healthier, younger-looking skin at any age. This means improved appearance, whether you're recovering from a skin injury or simply looking to improve your baseline glow.

---

85 Emília de Abreu Chaves M, Rodrigues de Araújo A, Piancastelli ACC, and Pinotti M. "Effects of low-power light therapy on wound healing: LASER x LED." An Bras Dermatol. 2014 Jul-Aug; 89(4): 616–623.

86 Wunsch A and Matuschka K. "A Controlled Trial to Determine the Efficacy of Red and Near-Infrared Light Treatment in Patient Satisfaction, Reduction of Fine Lines, Wrinkles, Skin Roughness, and Intradermal Collagen Density Increase." Photomedicine and Laser Surgery. Feb 2014; 32(2): 93-100.

87 Avci P, Gupta A, et al. Low-level laser (light) therapy (LLLT) in skin: stimulating, healing, restoring. Seminars in Cutaneous Medicine and Surgery. Mar 2013; 32(1): 41-52.

One 2017 study analyzed women aged 30-55 who used red light therapy on their faces. The research team found that red light therapy had a positive effect on the moisture content of skin, and diminished the appearance of wrinkles.[88]

These effects have made light therapy very popular with skincare professionals like estheticians and dermatologists.

Red light therapy is often used by doctors and hospitals to speed healing after major skin injuries such as burns and non-healing wounds. Now these benefits are available to you in your own home or local OsteoStrong clinic, through high-quality Joovv devices.

Shani Darden is one of the most respected skincare professionals in Hollywood, with A-list clients like Jessica Alba. She has a few things to say about red light therapy:

> *"Red light therapy is one of the best tools for naturally improving skin tone & texture and reducing fine lines & wrinkles. If you want to look younger and feel better, I can't recommend Joovv enough."*

Natural light is a powerful healing tool for your sleep, your skin, chronic pain, athletic training, and your skeletal system alike.

Improving Brain Health and Cognitive Function

It's easy to understand how natural light affects the skin at the surface of our bodies, where our mitochondria can be exposed to it directly. But researchers have also found that near-infrared light, including red light wavelengths, can penetrate deeper. When administered correctly these can reach bones, joints, and even the tissues of the brain.

When near-infrared light is applied directly to the head, wave-

---

88 Kim HK, Choi JH. Effects of radiofrequency, electroacupuncture, and low-level laser therapy on the wrinkles and moisture content of the forehead, eyes, and cheek. Journal of Physical Therapy Science. 2017 February.

lengths are able to pass through the skull and reach the brain to stimulate, preserve, and regenerate cells & tissues.

As world-famous cognitive coach Jim Kwik puts it: "We absorb light and use it as fuel for our bodies."

Jim is a learning expert who helps people across the world improve their memory, recall, and retention. He has started adding Joovv's light therapy treatments to his clients' cognitive health training and has seen great results.

Mr. Kwik himself uses light therapy daily to ensure that his brain functions at peak capacity. He believes it's one of the most powerful brain boosts available today.

The cognitive benefits of red-light therapy extend far beyond promoting circadian rhythm and healthy sleep, though getting sufficient sleep alone can boost learning and memory by 20-25%.

Building on a base of positive studies in laboratory animals, the first human trial of red-light therapy for cognitive performance showed big improvements in humans as well. Researchers found that people treated with red light therapy had significantly improved reaction times, better memory, and more sustained positive emotional states.[89]

Red light therapy has also been found to improve executive function - our ability to use higher brain functions such as attention, choice, and conscious control of our behavior.

Researchers found that people who received red light therapy treatments made fewer errors in sorting tests, which are tests designed to confuse users. The results of this 2017 study were very promising, as the authors believe results show that red light therapy may have exciting potential for treating or preventing memory loss from neuropsychological disorders or normal aging.[90]

---

89 Barrett DW, et al. Transcranial infrared laser stimulation produces beneficial cognitive and emotional effects in humans. 2013 Jan 29;230:13-23.
90 Blanco NJ, Maddox WT, Gonzalez-Lima F. Improving executive function

One of the most promising possibilities of red-light therapy is the treatment of Alzheimer's Disease and dementia.

Two of the first human trials of the use of red-light therapy in Alzheimer's Disease and dementia were published in 2017. Researchers found significant improvement in patients' executive function, clock drawing, memory, visual attention, immediate recall, and task switching. Researchers hope that these results can inject some optimism into a field that currently has few effective long-term treatments.[9192]

Even patients with traumatic brain injury (TBI) have responded positively to light therapy, showing improvements in mood and sleep. Scans have shown that light therapy helps regenerate damaged brain tissues and can play a big role in promoting neurogenesis - the creation of new brain cells and tissues.[939495]

The brain is extremely complex, and our understanding of its function lags well behind other areas of the body. But the early

---

using transcranial infrared laser stimulation. Journal of Neuropsychology. 2017 Mar;11(1):14-25.

91 Berman MH, Halper JP, Nichols TW, et al. Photobiomodulation with Near Infrared Light Helmet in a Pilot, Placebo Controlled Clinical Trial in Dementia Patients Testing Memory and Cognition. J Neurol Neurosci. 2017;8(1).

92Saltmarche AE, et al. Significant Improvement in Cognition in Mild to Moderately Severe Dementia Cases Treated with Transcranial Plus Intranasal Photobiomodulation; Case Series Report. Photomed Laser Surg. 2017 Aug;35(8):432-441.

93Joao S., Wellington P., Manoel T. "Transcranial light-emitting diode therapy for neuropsychological improvement after traumatic brain injury: new perspective for diffuse axonal lesion management" Medical Devices (Auckland, N.Z.). 2018; 11:139-146. dio: 10.2147/MDER.S155356

94 Michael H. "Shining light on the head: Photobiomodulation for brain disorders" BBA Clinical. 2016, December; 6: 113-124. dio: 10.1016/j. bbacli.2016.09.002

95Christopher T., Jeneita B., Matthew B., Likang X. "Traumatic Brain Injury - Related Emergency Department Visits, Hospitalizations, and Deaths - United States, 2007 and 2013" Center for Disease Control and Prevention. 2017, March; 66(9); 1-16.

indications from research and daily light therapy users like Jim Kwik are that it can have a major positive effect on cognition and brain cells.

Hormone Regulation with Red Light

Like inflammation and joint pain, tens of millions of Americans struggle with their thyroid and other hormone levels. These hormone imbalances can be influenced by artificial light, and can have a huge range of health consequences.

Millions of people take drugs like levothyroxine to regulate their hormone levels, and this usually ends up becoming a permanent solution. This approach simply replaces the body's ability to create thyroid instead of healing the body's natural thyroid gland production.

A 3-year study conducted by Brazilian researchers of people with chronic hypothyroidism and thyroiditis who take levothyroxine found improvements for those using light therapy to regulate hormone health.[96]

Researchers found that people with a history of taking levothyroxine were able to significantly reduce their doses after adding red light therapy to their routines. In nearly half of the cases patients were able to entirely stop taking the medication after extended red light therapy use.

More trials on red light therapy and hormone health are underway. One major focus is on thyroid function, as the health and function of the thyroid gland has a far-reaching impact on health and quality of life.

One health leader who has shared her success with Joovv and

---

96 Hofling DB, Chavantes MC, et al. Low-level laser in the treatment of patients with hypothyroidism induced by chronic autoimmune thyroiditis: a randomized, placebo-controlled clinical trial. Lasers in Surgery and Medicine. May 2013; 28(3): 743-53.

hormone regulation is Katie Wells, founder of the popular website Wellness Mama. She has long documented her battle with Hashimoto's Thyroiditis - an autoimmune attack on the thyroid gland - and how difficult it can be to raise young kids while fighting a thyroid condition.

Like millions of Americans, Katie has taken thyroid hormone medicine for many years. Seeking a more effective alternative with fewer side effects, she tried Joovv red light therapy.

Since beginning daily, full-body light therapy, Katie says she has been able to gradually lower her dose of thyroid medication over time, with noticeable improvements in general health, energy, and inflammation. Ms. Wells has also experienced improvement of her chronic thyroiditis symptoms, including less joint pain.

What to Look for in Your Own Light Therapy Device

OsteoStrong trusts Joovv for light therapy because it's the industry standard and has proven results across a wide range of benefits.

There are numerous options on the market if you're looking for a device for your own home. When shopping around, make sure to remember these key factors to get the best light therapy experience possible.

More Surface Area = More Benefit

No matter how big you happen to be, light therapy works better with a larger device that can cover more of your body with natural light at one time.

Coverage is key for light therapy because the magnitude of its overall health benefits depends on the percentage of your body's surface area that gets to enjoy the benefit of red light absorption. Smaller devices are unlikely to be able to mimic the effect of a large, whole-body device.

Shining red and near infrared light on just your wrist, for example, may help reduce inflammation and pain in that area. But it's not likely to impact your whole body and lead to system-wide decreased inflammation or increased energy.

When you use a device that's large enough to cover your whole body, millions of cells can take in natural light at once and start producing energy for your body. Uniform coverage is key for optimal results, and a small device that covers only a portion of your body will not provide you with the best health benefits. So if you want optimal treatments, look for a bigger device, even if it costs more.

Targeted light therapy treatments can work well for specific target areas like a scar, the skin on your face, or an inflamed ankle. But for the range of full-body benefits, you need to bask your body in more light.

Look For a Higher Total Power Level

Measuring the power of light is a complex business, and it's nearly impossible to get accurate readings yourself without investing in expensive diagnostic equipment. Devices commonly measure power in terms of irradiance, or the amount of power being delivered by light hitting the surface area of the instrument.

The problem with this is, your body is typically larger than the measurement instrument. And the question you are interested in is the total amount of light being put out by the device and falling on your body; not just the amount of light hitting the small area you are measuring.

Because getting full-body treatment is so vital, you have to go further and measure total light output based on both the power per unit of surface area, and the total area the device covers. The key measurement isn't just how much power a device can produce in one small area, but rather how much energy it can deliver to your whole body.

That's how photobiomodulation scientists like Dr. Michael

Hamblin of Harvard Medical School measure light therapy devices. Dr. Hamblin is one of the leading light therapy researchers in the world, and he says this about power measurements:

"Total light energy is the most accurate and comprehensive way to measure the power of light therapy devices and treatments. If you only account for irradiance—versus how much total energy a device delivers—you miss the larger picture of how light therapy positively benefits the person using it."

The manufacturer of a small device may advertise their high power, based on a high irradiance number. But that measurement may have been taken over only a tiny area, measured by a small instrument. This misses the point of light therapy. A larger device with more coverage will deliver far more power and greater biological effect because it affects more cells at one time.

Smaller devices with targeted treatments often lack the requisite power to produce clinical health results. A high-quality LED light therapy device should deliver a dose of at least 15-20 joules/cm^2.

If you're aiming for full-body light therapy—which is optimal— look for a total energy output of at least 200,000 joules total.

Know Your Wavelengths

A Joovv device delivers wavelengths of red and near infrared natural light in the mid-600 and mid-800 nanometer range. As you may have gathered, those numbers are important.[97]

We've already mentioned that all the clinical trials showing benefits use red and near-infrared wavelengths, while blue light can actually be disruptive to your circadian rhythm and overall health.

Sunlight contains a wide spectrum of colors and wavelengths, including invisible wavelengths like ultraviolet and near-infrared

---

97 de Almeida P1, Lopes-Martins RA, De Marchi T, et al. "Red (660 nm) and infrared (830 nm) low-level laser therapy in skeletal muscle fatigue in humans: what is better?" Lasers Med Sci. 2012 Mar;27(2):453-8.

light. Obviously, the effects of these two wavelengths are not the same: near-infrared wavelengths stimulate skin cells to heal and grow, while ultraviolet wavelengths damage DNA and can cause sunburns and cancers.

Most clinical research has found that red and near infrared light are the most effective wavelengths for health benefits. This means that these are the wavelengths you want in your red light therapy device.

You don't want a device that produces potentially harmful wavelengths, such as blue and ultraviolet light. You also don't want a device that gets much of its power from "junk wavelengths" - wavelengths that won't really make a physiological difference in your body.

One important "junk wavelength" range to be aware of is the 700s nm range. Although these wavelengths are close to the mid-600 and mid-800 nm ranges that are beneficial, these middle ranges have not been found to have strong clinical effects.

Red and near infrared light is consistently found to work best for people, so avoid products that include wavelengths in the 700s nm scale. These wavelengths are fillers that may boost a device's apparent power on the irradiance scale while not doing anything for your body.

Quality Control for Light Therapy

When choosing your light therapy device, look for a manufacturer that insists on quality. Policies like good customer service and warranties are good indicators of device quality, as manufacturers are unlikely to provide these for devices that they know are low-quality.

Too many light therapy brands sell devices online, but don't back them up with warrantees or offer resources to new users. The best brands will also provide the public with plenty of educational resources about the science and technology behind their product.

Any company can market a device online and claim that it has certain effects, but the more reliable manufacturers will be transparent with information like clinical data from studies and trials.

Light for A Modern World, Through OsteoStrong Clinics

At OsteoStrong, we strive to offer the most effective biohacking technologies to our users at accessible prices. That's why we offer our exclusive, patented Spectrum robotic osteogenic loading devices, high-quality PEMF devices, cutting edge light therapy, and vibration plates for neural and growth hormone activation.

Light therapy is one of the most promising health interventions available today. With its underlying mechanism of action being so new to science, we are just beginning to explore the potential of this technology. The results of clinical trials so far tell us that the potential is real: we just need to discover exactly how far it goes.

From professional athletes and trainers to celebrity estheticians and dermatologists, professionals across disciplines are using light therapy treatments to obtain better health and better performance for their clients. Scientists and stars alike are seeing results from this technology.

At OsteoStrong, we're excited to offer Joovv red light therapy devices so our members can enjoy these natural health benefits as well.

OsteoStrong trusts Joovv in our centers because they've proven themselves to be the industry standard for light therapy, and the one manufacturer that's really driving innovation and education in the field.

Joovv is doing this both by creating the most effective light therapy products on the market, and by partnering with leading medical researchers & clinics around the world. Joovv is actively engaged in researching & testing the possibilities & applications of light therapy science.

We hope you'll take advantage of red-light therapy technology the next time you stop into one of our OsteoStrong clinics.

CHAPTER 6

Biohack Your Lifestyle
Kyle Zagrodzky

We live in an era of unprecedented possibilities. With cutting-edge scientific advancements at our fingertips, we can heal and augment our bodies' capabilities faster than ever before.

All of the technologies discussed in this book convey profound benefits that can change the lives of most people. But as we've already seen, *how* you use them will determine what results you get, and how fast.

We also recognize that it might not be practical for all of our readers to adopt all of these technologies, as many U.S. cities do not yet have OsteoStrong locations where many of these technologies are provided all in one place on an affordable basis.

So how do you decide which of these techniques and technologies to prioritize in your own life? And if you choose one, which *variant* or method of using it will be best for you?

What Is Your Goal?

All good biohackers know to ask one question before creating their strategy for success: what is my *goal?* You cannot find the shortest, easiest route to your destination, after all, unless you know where you are going.

This book has two main target audiences: those seeking to recover from disease or poor health, and those seeking to push their mental and physical abilities into superhuman realms.

Some of our readers might fall into *both* groups. After all, we've now seen that growth and strength are not actually restricted to our younger years, as was once believed. With the help of cutting-edge science, an ambitious retiree can easily surpass their twenty-something self in physical and mental prowess.

Because recovering a baseline level of health is necessary *before* starting a routine to surpass normal human capabilities, we'll start with recommendations for those whose quality of life is currently impaired by pain, exhaustion, or medical conditions.

Recovering Health

Many of the authors included in this manuscript met through their shared goal of fighting osteoporosis. As you've seen, OsteoStrong's osteogenic loading devices were originally designed to do just that, and PEMF and red light therapy have also shown remarkable clinical results in the same battle against dangerously low bone density.

Remember that osteogenic loading can also provide enormous relief for back and joint pain, so if chronic pain is a major factor holding you back, you may wish to push osteogenic loading to the top of your list even if your bone density is good. OsteoStrong's PEMF and red light therapy offerings offer a triple threat, soothing and improving chronic pain through several different physiological mechanisms.

It's amazing how much the simple act of relieving pain can

increase your ability to build strength, eat a healthy diet, and live a joyful life.

In addition to strengthening your musculoskeletal system and relieving pain through osteogenic loading, you can also take advantage of the gentle yet transformative PEMF and red light therapy treatments offered at many OsteoStrong locations.

The combination of safe, controlled, low-impact osteogenic loading, circulation and oxygenation-enhancing PEMF devices, and energizing and revitalizing red light treatments can't be beat for people looking to restore health and strength at any age.

Biohacking Your Brain

Once you are comfortable with your basic level of health, you may prioritize biohacking your body, or your brain. For some people, athletic performance is their number one priority. For others, it's having the energy and clarity to deliver supercharged performances in business, academics, or family life.

If mental clarity, exercise, and reliable mental performance are your goals then red light therapy for sleep and brain stimulation is your best friend. You may even wish to consider purchasing a device for your home so that you can enjoy its benefits daily and target your brain activity specifically.

PEMF devices found at OsteoStrong centers can also help to improve mood and increase blood circulation to your brain, and osteogenic loading can be used to approve your overall metabolism by helping your body metabolize calories more efficiently.

Remember that adequate sleep improves learning and memory by 20-25% - not to mention its effect on mood, energy levels, and on overall physical health through our stress hormone systems. Many Americans underestimate the importance of sleep, or don't even realize that they're sleeping poorly until they experience restorative sleep for the first time in months or years.

Biohacking Your Body

The traditional view of the "superhuman" individual is someone with bulging muscles and incredible strength. We're all for that!

Every athlete knows that exercise is the way to gain a stronger body. But as you've learned here, there are modes of exercise available that act as accelerators to the results many you may be seeking.

Muscle strength is limited by bone strength, so it's wise to include osteogenic loading in your muscle-building or strength training workout if at all possible. In addition to strengthening your bones, osteogenic loading provides some direct strength gain by loading your body in a way that is similar to what's experienced in high-weight, low-repetition weight lifting and other high-impact activities.

Once your bones are strong enough to accomodate remarkable force, you can continue supercharging your strength growth through the use of osteogenic loading to stimulate the formation of new myosin in your muscle cells.

If you're shooting for superhuman strength, you'll likely take advantage of both biohacking and traditional modes of weightlifting and training. But don't forget to stop into your local OsteoStrong clinic for a red light therapy session after each intense training session - this will assure that you gain strength and performance faster and recover more quickly so you can go back out there and train again.

You Can Have It All

Remember, none of the goals above are mutually exclusive. It's possible (and fun!) to build a lifestyle which optimizes your health, brain function, and physical strength all at once.

The suggestions above are simply a "starter kit." Biohacking approaches to strength and wellness often work best when used in combination with traditional approaches. The brain-and body-enhancing effects of the technology we've discussed here form a wonderful synergy with traditional diet, exercise, and medical treatment to produce results much faster and with greater ease than traditional techniques alone.

You may very well find that, as you attain one goal, another starts to look more feasible or appealing to you. Maybe something that once seemed out of reach now seems achievable.

And that is the beauty of this work. There's no reason to ever stop getting better.

ABOUT THE AUTHORS

John Jaquish, PhD

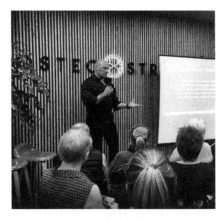

John Jaquish, PhD, is the inventor of the most effective bone density building medical device, which has reversed osteoporosis for thousands and created more powerful and fracture-resistant athletes.

His devices have been placed in over 300 clinics worldwide. Osteogenic loading has now helped well over 20,000 individuals to improve their bone health.

Dr. Jaquish is a research professor at Rushmore University, speaks at scientific conferences all over the world, has been featured on many of the top health podcasts, is an editor of multiple medical journals, and is a nominee of the National Medal of Science.

Kyle Zagrodzky

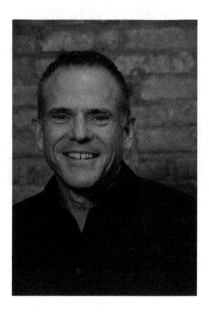

Kyle Zagrodzky is Founder and CEO of OsteoStrong, the health and wellness system that provides musculoskeletal strength conditioning in less than 10 minutes per week using patented and scientifically proven osteogenic loading robotic devices.

OsteoStrong introduced new possibilities in modern fitness and aging prevention in 2012. It has since helped thousands of clients between ages 8 and 92 improve strength, balance, endurance and bone density.

Greg Musser, ND

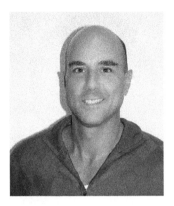

Dr. Greg Musser is the President of Swiss Bionic Solutions USA and has held the position since 2012. Swiss Bionic Solutions is the leader in pulsed magnetic field medical equipment manufacturing and distribution.

Greg earned his Doctorate in Naturopathy from Trinity School of Natural Health. He focused his study on bio-electromagnetics, which deals with the interactions of electromagnetic fields and biological systems.

Over the past year, along with Greg's naturopathic education, Swiss Bionic Solutions has sent him to Washington, D.C, where he has been involved with the Advanced Medical Technology Association (AdvaMed) to further SBS's mission of educating the public and promoting pulsed magnetic fields for home use.

Scott Nelson

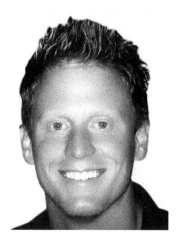

Scott Nelson is a medtech enthusiast, ambitious doer, and curious by nature. He has held sales and marketing leadership roles for some of the largest medical device companies in the world including Medtronic, Covidien, Boston Scientific, C.R. Bard, and ConMed.

Scott founded Medsider.com in 2010 with one simple goal: Help ambitious doers learn from experienced medtech thought leaders. Scott's work with Medsider has been featured in publications like Forbes, Mass Device, MedCity News, and MD +DI. On a monthly basis, tens of thousands of people listen to Scott's interviews with medtech experts.

Scott cofounded Joovv in 2015 and is currently focused on commercializing the first professional-grade, full-body red light therapy system with a patented, modular design. In addition, he's also an advisor to the Medical Devices Group, which includes over 300,000 members worldwide. He graduated with a B.A. in Biology from Grand View University.

REFERENCES & RESOURCES

1. Deere, K., Sayers, A., Rittweger, J., & Tobias, J. H. (2012). Habitual levels of high, but not moderate or low, impact activity are positively related to hip BMD and geometry: results from a population-based study of adolescents. Journal of bone and mineral research, 27(9), 1887-1895.

2. Leblanc, A., Schneider, V., Evans, H., Engelbretson, D., & Krebs, J. (1990). Bone mineral loss and recovery after 17 weeks of bed rest. Journal of Bone and Mineral Research. 5,8. 1523-4681.

3. Marcus, R. (1996). Skeletal "impact" of exercise. The Lancet, 348(9038), 1326-1327.

4. Surgeon General (2004). Bone health and osteoporosis: A report of the Surgeon General. Rockville, MD. . U.S. Dept. of Health and Human Services, Public Health Service, Office of the Surgeon General ; Washington, D.C.: U.S. G.P.O., 2004. p.436, 223.

5. Mookerjee, S., & Ratamess N. (1999). Comparison of Strength Differences and Joint Action Durations Between Full and Partial Range-of-Motion Bench Press Exercise. Journal of Strength and Conditioning Research, 1999,

13(1), 76–81 1999 National Strength & Conditioning Association.

6. Jaquish, J. (2013). Multiple-of-bodyweight axial bone loading using novel exercise intervention with and without bisphosphonate use for osteogenic adaptation. Osteoporosis International. 198; 24(4), s594-s595.

7. Hunte, B., Jaquish, J., & Huck, C. (2015). Axial Bone Osteogenic Loading-Type Resistance Therapy Showing BMD and Functional Bone Performance Musculoskeletal Adaptation Over 24 Weeks with Postmenopausal Female Subjects. Journal of Osteoporosis & Physical Activity, 3(146), 2.

8. Ferguson, B. (2014). ACSM's guidelines for exercise testing and prescription 9th Ed. 2014. The Journal of the Canadian Chiropractic Association, 58(3), 328.

9. Bawin SM and Adey WR. 1976. Sensitivity of calcium binding in cerebral tissue to weak environmental electric fields oscillating at low frequency. Proc Natl Acad Sci U S A. 1976 Jun; 73(6): 1999–2003.

10. McKay JC, Prato FS, et al. A literature review: the effects of magnetic field exposure on blood flow and blood vessels in the microvasculature. Bioelectromagnetics. 2007 Feb;28(2):81-98.

11. Muehsam D, Lalezari P, et al. Non-thermal radio-frequency and static magnetic fields increase rate of hemoglobin deoxygenation in a cell-free preparation. PLOS One. 2013 Apr 12;8(4):e61752.

12. Jerabek J, Pawluk W. Magnetic therapy in Eastern Europe:

a review of 30 years of research. Publ Advanced Magnetic Research of the Delaware Valley, Chicago, 1996.

13. Warmke U. Survey of some working mechanisms of pulsating electromagnetic fields PEMF). Bioelectrochem Bioeneg 27(3):317-320,1992.

14. Victoria G, Petrisor B, Drew B, et al. 2009. Bone stimulation for fracture healing: What's all the fuss? Indian J Orthop 2009; 43:117-120.

15. Gorissen BM, Wolschrijn CF, van Vilsteren AA, et al. 2016. Trabecular bone of precocials at birth; Are they prepared to run for the wolf(f)? J Morphol 2016; 277:948-956.

16. The classic: Fundamental aspects of fracture treatment by Iwao Yasuda, reprinted from J. Kyoto Med. Soc., 4: 395-406, 1953. Clin Orthop Relat Res 1977 5-8.

17. Schemitsch E, Kuzyk P. The science of electrical stimulation therapy for fracture healing. *Indian Journal of Orthopaedics*. 2009;43(2):127. doi:10.4103/0019-5413.50846.

18. Bassett CA, Mitchell SN, Norton L, et al. 1978. Repair of non-unions by pulsing electromagnetic fields. Acta Orthop Belg 1978; 44:706-724.

19. Gupta AK, Srivastava KP, Avasthi S. 2009. Pulsed electromagnetic stimulation in nonunion of tibial diaphyseal fractures. Indian J Orthop 2009; 43:156-160.

20. Meskens MW, Stuyck JA, Feys H, et al. 1990. Treatment of nonunion using pulsed electromagnetic fields: a retrospective follow-up study. Acta Orthop Belg 1990; 56:483-488.

21. Assiotis A, Sachinis NP, Chalidis BE. 2012. Pulsed electromagnetic fields for the treatment of tibial delayed unions

and nonunions. A prospective clinical study and review of the literature. J Orthop Surg Res 2012; 7:24.

22. Kuzyk PR, Schemitsch EH. 2009. The science of electrical stimulation therapy for fracture healing. Indian J Orthop 2009; 43:127-131.

23. Chalidis B, Sachinis N, Assiotis A, et al. 2011. Stimulation of bone formation and fracture healing with pulsed electromagnetic fields: biologic responses and clinical implications. Int J Immunopathol Pharmacol 2011; 24:17-20.

24. Gupta AK, Srivastava KP, Avasthi S. 2009. Pulsed electromagnetic stimulation in nonunion of tibial diaphyseal fractures. Indian J Orthop 2009; 43:156-160.

25. Meskens MW, Stuyck JA, Feys H, et al. 1990. Treatment of nonunion using pulsed electromagnetic fields: a retrospective follow-up study. Acta Orthop Belg 1990; 56:483-488.

26. Hannemann PF, Mommers EH, Schots JP, et al. 2014. The effects of low-intensity pulsed ultrasound and pulsed electromagnetic fields bone growth stimulation in acute fractures: a systematic review and meta-analysis of randomized controlled trials. Arch Orthop Trauma Surg 2014; 134;1093-1106

27. Dhawan SK, Conti SF, Towers J, et al. 2004. The effect of pulsed electromagnetic fields on hindfoot arthrodesis: a prospective study. J Foot Ankle Surg 2004; 43:93-96.

28. Bassett CA, Mitchell SN, Gaston SR. 1981. Treatment of ununited tibial diaphyseal fractures with pulsing electromagnetic fields. J Bone Joint Surg Am 1981; 63:511-523.

29. de Haas WG, Watson J, Morrison DM. 1980. Non-invasive

treatment of ununited fractures of the tibia using electrical stimulation. J Bone Joint Surg Br 1980; 62-B:465-470.

30. Nelson FR, Brighton CT, Ryaby J, et al. 2003. Use of physical forces in bone healing. J Am Acad Orthop Surg 2003; 11:344-354.

31. Zhou W, Yu L, Fan J, et al. 2017. Endogenous Parathyroid Hormone Promotes Fracture Healing by Increasing Expression of BMPR2 through cAMP/PKA/CREB Pathway in Mice. Cell Physiol Biochem 2017; 42:551-563.

32. Pai MV. 2017. Osteoporosis Prevention and Management. J Obstet Gynaecol India 2017; 67:237-242.

33. Golob AL, Laya MB. 2015. Osteoporosis: screening, prevention, and management. Med Clin North Am 2015; 99:587-606.

34. Verbovoy AF, Pashentseva AV, Sharonova LA. 2017. Osteoporosis: Current state of the art. Ter Arkh 2017; 89:90-97.

35. Ensrud KE, Crandall CJ. 2017. Osteoporosis. Ann Intern Med 2017; 167:ITC17-ITC32.

36. Watts NB, Bilezikian JP, Camacho PM, et al. 2010. American Association of Clinical Endocrinologists Medical Guidelines for Clinical Practice for the diagnosis and treatment of postmenopausal osteoporosis. Endocr Pract 2010; 16:S1-37.

37. Eyres KS, Saleh M, Kanis JA. 1996. Effect of pulsed electromagnetic fields on bone formation and bone loss during limb lengthening. Bone 1996; 18:505-509.

38. Rubin CT, McLeod KJ, Lanyon LE. 1989. Prevention of osteoporosis by pulsed electromagnetic fields. J Bone Joint Surg Am 1989; 71:411-417.

39. Tabrah F, Hoffmeier M, Bassett CA, et al. 1990. Bone

density changes in osteoporosis-prone women exposed to pulsed electromagnetic fields (PEMFs). J Bone Miner Res 1990; 5:437-442.

40. Garland DE, Adkins RH, Matsuno NN, et al. 1999. The effect of pulsed electromagnetic fields on osteoporosis at the knee in individuals with spinal cord injury. J Spinal Cord Med 1999; 22:239-245.

41. Liu H, Liu Y, Yang L, et al. 2014. Curative effects of pulsed electromagnetic fields on postmenopausal osteoporosis. Sheng Wu Yi Xue Gong Cheng Xue Za Zhi 2014; 31:48-52.

42. Wang R, Wu H, Yang Y, et al. 2016. Effects of electromagnetic fields on osteoporosis: A systematic literature review. Electromagn Biol Med 2016; 35:384-390.

43. Weng YX, Gao QY, Shao HWy, et al. 2003. Osteoporosis pain and effectiveness of pulsed electromagnetic fields in treating pain in patients with osteoporosis. Chin J Osteoporos (China)2003; 9:3-17.

44. Hayashi Y. 2007. Bone diseases with Pain. Osteoporosis. Clin Calcium 2007; 17:606-612.

45. Verbovoy AF, Pashentseva AV, Sharonova LA. 2017. Osteoporosis. Current state of the art. Ter Arkh 2017; 89:90-97.

46. Ensrud KE, Crandall CJ. 2017. Osteoporosis. Ann Intern Med 2017; 167:ITC17-ITC32.

47. Fang QQ, Li ZZ, Zhou J, et al. 2016. Low-frequency pulsed electromagnetic fields promotes rat osteoblast differentiation in vitro through cAMP/PKA signal pathway. Nan Fang Yi Ke Da Xue Xue Bao 2016; 36:1508-1513.

48. Liu HF, Yang L, He HC, et al. 2013. Pulsed electromagnetic fields on postmenopausal osteoporosis in Southwest

China: a randomized, active-controlled clinical trial. Bio-electromagnetics 2013; 34:323-332.

49. Liu H, Yang L, He H, et al. 2013. The hemorheological safety of pulsed electromagnetic fields in postmenopausal women with osteoporosis in southwest China: a random-ized, placebo controlled clinical trial. Clin Hemorheol Microcirc 2013; 55:285-295.

50. Part III: Pain Terms, A Current List with Definitions and Notes on Usage. Classification of Chronic Pain, Second Edition, IASP Task Force on Taxonomy, edited by H. Merskey and N. Bogduk, IASP Press, Seattle, 1994, pp 209-214.

51. Jerabek, J and Pawluk, W. Magnetic therapy in Eastern Europe: a review of 30 years of research. Publ. Advanced Magnetic Research of the Delaware Valley, Chicago, 1996.

52. Trock DH. Electromagnetic fields and magnets. Investi-gational treatment for musculoskeletal disorders. Rheum Dis Clin North Am 2000 Feb;26(1):51-62, viii.

53. Preszler, RR. A non-invasive complementary method of reducing chronic muscular low back pain using perma-nent magnetic therapy. A Thesis For the degree of Masters in Physician Assistant Studies University of Nebraska School of Medicine, Physician Assistant Program, Lin-coln, Nebraska, 2000.

54. Rauscher E, Van Bise W. L. Pulsed magnetic field treat-ment of chronic back pain. Bioelectromagnetics Society, 23rd Annual Meeting, St. Paul, MN, June,2001.

55. Thuile C, Walzl M. Evaluation of electromagnetic fields in the treatment of pain in patients with lumbar radicu-

lopathy or the whiplash syndrome. NeuroRehabilitation 2002; 17: 63-67.

56. Mitbreit IM, Savchenko AG, et al. Low-frequency magnetic field in the complex treatment of patients with lumbar osteochondrosis. Ortop Travmatol Protez (10):24-27, 1986.

57. Prusinski A, Wielka J, Durko A. Pulsating electromagnetic field in the therapy of headache. J Bioelectr 7(1):127-128 Second Symposium on Magnetotherapy, Szekesfehervar, Hungary, May, 1987.

58. Sherman, R. A.; Acosta, N. M.; Robson, L. Treatment of migraine with pulsing electromagnetic fields: a double-blind, placebo-controlled study. Headache 39(8):567-575, 1999.

59. Foley-Nolan, D.; Barry, C.; Coughlan, R. J.; O'Connor, P.; Roden, D. Pulsed high frequency (27 mhz) electromagnetic therapy for persistent neck pain. A double blind, placebo-controlled study of 20 patients. Orthopedics 13(4):445-451, 1990.

60. Kjellman GV, Skargren EI, Oberg BE. A critical analysis of randomised clinical trials on neck pain and treatment efficacy. A review of the literature. Scand J Rehabil Med 31(3):139-152, 1999.

61. Stewart DJ, Stewart JE. Acta Med Hung 1989;46(4):323-37. The destabilization of an abnormal physiological balanced situation, chronic musculoskeletal pain, utilizing magnetic biological device.

62. Kobinger W, Fischer G, et al. Using Magnetic Fields to Increase Flexibility and Reduce Pain with Respect to Ail-

ments of the Ambulatory Apparatus. 26th Conference of the Austrian Society for Internal Medicine. July 1995.

63. Pujol J, Pascual-Leone A, et al. The effect of repetitive magnetic stimulation on localized musculoskeletal pain. Neuroreport 9(8):1745-1748, 1998.

64. Thomas AW, Prato FS. Magnetic field based pain therapeutics and diagnostics. Bioelectromagnetics Society, 24th Annual Meeting, Quebec City, PQ, Canada, June, 2002.

65. Ghione S, Luschi P, et al. Electromagnetic fields and nociception: physiological and clinical responses. Forum on Future European Research on Mobile Communications and Health, Bordeaux, France, April, 1999.

66. Sartucci F, Bonfiglio L, et al. Changes in pain perception and pain-related somatosensory evoked potentials in humans produced by exposure to oscillating magnetic fields. Brain Res 769(2):362-366, 1997.

67. Fleming, JL, Persinger, MA, et al. Magnetic pulses elevate nociceptive thresholds: comparisons with opiate receptor compounds in normal and seizure-induced brain-damaged rats. Electro Magnetobiol 13(1):67-75, 1994.

68. Hutchinson D, Witt S, Fairpo CG. Pulsed electromagnetic energy therapy in third molar surgery. Oral Surg Oral Med Oral Pathol, 46(6):748-754, 1978.

69. Tesic D, Djuric M, et al. PEMF aided pain reduction in stomatology. Bioelectromagnetics Society, 21st Annual Meeting, Long Beach, CA, Abstract, June, 1999.

70. Schroter M. Conservative Treatment of 240 Patients with Magnetic Field Therapy. Medizinisch- Orthopadische Technik. March/April 1976 (2):78.

71. Markov MS, Pilla A. A. Electromagnetic field stimulation

of soft tissue: pulsed radiofrequency treatment of post-operative pain and edema. Wounds 7(4):143-151, 1995.

72. Jacobson JL, Gorman R, Yamanashi WS, et al. Low-amplitude, extremely low frequency magnetic fields for the treatment of osteoarthritic knees: a double-blind clinical study. Altern Ther Health Med 7(5):54-60, 62-64, 66-69, 2001.

73. Pawluk W, Turk Z, et al. Treatment of osteoarthritis with a new broadband PEMF signal. Bioelectromagnetics Society, 24th Annual Meeting, Quebec City, QC, Canada, June, 2002.

74. Kusaka C, Seto A, et al. Pulse magnetic treatment and whole-body, alternating current magnetic treatment for post-herpetic neuralgia. J Jpn Biomagnetism Bioelectromagnetics Soc 8(2):29-38, 1995.

75. Munglani R. The longer term effect of pulsed radiofrequency for neuropathic pain. Pain 80(1-2):437-439, 1999.

76. Rehacek J, Straub J, Benova H. The effect of magnetic fields on coxarthroses. Fysiatr Revmatol Vestn 60(2):66-68, 1982.

77. Cieslar G, Sieron A, Radelli J. The estimation of therapeutic effect of variable magnetic fields in patients with diabetic neuropathy including vibratory sensibility. Balneol Pol, 1995, 37(1): 23-27.

78. Jerabek J, Pawluk W. Magnetic therapy in Eastern Europe: a review of 30 years of research. Publ Advanced Magnetic Research of the Delaware Valley, Chicago, 1996.

79. Klepeis N., Nelson W., Ott W., Robinson J., Tsang A., Switzer P., Behar J., Hern S., Engelmann W. "The National Human Activity Pattern Survey (NHAPS): a resource for

assessing exposure to environmental pollutants". Journal of Exposure Analysis and Environmental Epidemiology 2001;11, 231-252.

80. Hatori M., Gronfier C., Van Gelder R., Bernstein P., Carreras J., Panda S., Mark F., Silney D., Hunt C., Hirota T., Furukawa T., Tsubota K. "Global rise of potential health hazards caused by blue light-induced circadian disruption in modern aging societies". NPJ Aging Mech Dis. 2017; 3:9. doi: 10.1038/s41514-017-001-2.

81. Morita T., Tokura H. "Effects of lights of different color temperature on the nocturnal changes in core temperature and melatonin in humans" Journal of Physiological Anthropology. 1996, September; 15(5):243-246.

82. Loeb LM, Amorim RP, et al. "Botulinum toxin A (BT-A) versus low-level laser therapy (LLLT) in chronic migraine treatment: a comparison." Arquivos de neuro-psiquiatria. 2018 Oct;76(10):663-667.

83. Zhao J., Tian Y., Nie J., Xu J., Liu D. "Red light and the sleep quality and endurance performance of Chinese female basketball players" Journal of Athletic Training. 2012, November-December; 47(6):673-678. doi: 10.4085/1062-47.6.08.

84. Chang WD, Wu JH, et al. Therapeutic outcomes of low level laser therapy for closed bone fracture in the human wrist and hand. Photomedicine and Laser Surgery. 2014 April.

85. Michael R. Hamblin. "Mechanisms and applications of the anti-inflammatory effects of photobiomodulation." AIMS Biophys. 2017; 4(3): 337–361.

86. Ferraresi C, Bertucci D, Schiavinato J, et al. "Effects

of Light-Emitting Diode Therapy on Muscle Hypertrophy, Gene Expression, Performance, Damage, and Delayed-Onset Muscle Soreness: Case-control Study with a Pair of Identical Twins." Am J Phys Med Rehabil. 2016 Oct;95(10):746-57.

87. Borges LS, et al. Light-emitting diode phototherapy improves muscle recovery after a damaging exercise. Lasers in Medical Science. 2014 May;29(3):1139-44.

88. Brosseau L, Welch V, et al. Low level laser therapy for osteoarthritis and rheumatoid arthritis: a meta-analysis. The Journal of Rheumatology. Aug 2000; 27(8): 1961-9.

89. Dellagrana RA, Rossato M, et al. Photobiomodulation Therapy on Physiological and Performance Parameters During Running Tests: Dose-Response Effects. Journal of Strength and Conditioning Research. 2018 Oct;32(10):2807-2815.

90. Miranda EF, Tomazoni SS, et al. When is the best moment to apply photobiomodulation therapy (PBMT) when associated to a treadmill endurance-training program? A randomized, triple-blinded, placebo-controlled clinical trial. Lasers in Med Science. 2018 May;33(4):719-727.

91. Vanin AA, et al. What is the best moment to apply phototherapy when associated to a strength training program? A randomized, double-blinded, placebo-controlled trial : Phototherapy in association to strength training. Lasers in Medical Science. 2016 Nov;31(8):1555-1564.

92. Emília de Abreu Chaves M, Rodrigues de Araújo A, Piancastelli ACC, and Pinotti M. "Effects of low-power

light therapy on wound healing: LASER x LED." An Bras Dermatol. 2014 Jul-Aug; 89(4): 616–623.

93. Wunsch A and Matuschka K. "A Controlled Trial to Determine the Efficacy of Red and Near-Infrared Light Treatment in Patient Satisfaction, Reduction of Fine Lines, Wrinkles, Skin Roughness, and Intradermal Collagen Density Increase." Photomedicine and Laser Surgery. Feb 2014; 32(2): 93-100.

94. Avci P, Gupta A, et al. Low-level laser (light) therapy (LLLT) in skin: stimulating, healing, restoring. Seminars in Cutaneous Medicine and Surgery. Mar 2013; 32(1): 41-52.

95. Kim HK, Choi JH. Effects of radiofrequency, electroacupuncture, and low-level laser therapy on the wrinkles and moisture content of the forehead, eyes, and cheek. Journal of Physical Therapy Science. 2017 February.

96. Barrett DW, et al. Transcranial infrared laser stimulation produces beneficial cognitive and emotional effects in humans. 2013 Jan 29;230:13-23.

97. Blanco NJ, Maddox WT, Gonzalez-Lima F. Improving executive function using transcranial infrared laser stimulation Journal of Neuropsychology. 2017 Mar;11(1):14-25.

98. Berman MH, Halper JP, Nichols TW, et al. Photobiomodulation with Near Infrared Light Helmet in a Pilot, Placebo Controlled Clinical Trial in Dementia Patients Testing Memory and Cognition. J Neurol Neurosci. 2017;8(1).

99. Saltmarche AE, et al. Significant Improvement in Cognition in Mild to Moderately Severe Dementia Cases Treated with Transcranial Plus Intranasal Photobiomod-

ulation: Case Series Report. Photomed Laser Surg. 2017 Aug;35(8):432-441.

100. Joao S., Wellington P., Manoel T. "Transcranial light-emitting diode therapy for neuropsychological improvement after traumatic brain injury: new perspective for diffuse axonal lesion management" Medical Devices (Auckland, N.Z.). 2018; 11:139-146. dio: 10.2147/MDER.S155356.

101. Michael H. "Shining light on the head: Photobiomodulation for brain disorders" BBA Clinical. 2016, December; 6: 113-124. dio: 10.1016/j.bbacli.2016.09.002.

102. Christopher T., Jeneita B., Matthew B., Likang X. "Traumatic Brain Injury - Related Emergency Department Visits, Hospitalizations, and Deaths - United States, 2007 and 2013" Center for Disease Control and Prevention. 2017, March; 66(9); 1-16.

103. Hofling DB, Chavantes MC, et al. Low-level laser in the treatment of patients with hypothyroidism induced by chronic autoimmune thyroiditis: a randomized, placebo-controlled clinical trial. Lasers in Surgery and Medicine. May 2013; 28(3): 743-53.

104. de Almeida P1, Lopes-Martins RA, De Marchi T, et al. "Red (660 nm) and infrared (830 nm) low-level laser therapy in skeletal muscle fatigue in humans: what is better?" Lasers Med Sci. 2012 Mar;27(2):453-8.

Milton Keynes UK
Ingram Content Group UK Ltd.
UKHW021258081123
432199UK00016B/718